The Natural Path to Hormonal Wellness, Part 1

Katarina Nolte

The Natural Path to Hormonal Wellness, Part 1 by Katarina Nolte
Pages: 201 (23,609 words); Copyright © 2014 by Katarina Nolte.
All rights reserved. http://katarinanolte.com/ July 2014

DEDICATION

For P.

The Natural Path to Hormonal Wellness, Part 1 by Katarina Nolte
Pages: 201 (23,609 words); Copyright © 2014 by Katarina Nolte.
All rights reserved. http://katarinanolte.com/ July 2014

EPIGRAPH

Some consider the bio-availability of herbs extracted in tinctures superior to teas and decoctions. Maybe so, maybe not. But one thing's for sure, store bought tinctures are pricey. Even one ounce bottles go from ten to twenty U.S. dollars, depending on the herb type and quality. But you can make your own large volume tinctures easily and cheaply for long term cost efficient use with high quality ingredients of your choice. Thanks to the alcohol content, a large batch can last forever without losing potency.

Paul Fassa ~ Easily Make Your Own Herbal Tinctures And Save Money | Shift Frequency

http://www.shiftfrequency.com/paul-fassa-easily-make-your-own-herbal-tinctures-and-save-money/

The Natural Path to Hormonal Wellness, Part 1 by Katarina Nolte
Pages: 201 (23,609 words); Copyright © 2014 by Katarina Nolte.
All rights reserved. http://katarinanolte.com/ July 2014

TABLE OF CONTENTS

The Natural Path to Hormonal Wellness, Part 1 by Katarina Nolte
Pages: 201 (23,609 words); Copyright © 2014 by Katarina Nolte.
All rights reserved. http://katarinanolte.com/ July 2014

DISCLAIMER

The statements and information in this book have not been evaluated by the FDA. It is not intended to treat, diagnose, cure, mitigate or prevent any disease. The content provided is for informational purposes only. Before starting any health or wellness program always seek the advice of your physician or other qualified, licensed health professional. Neither the author nor publisher take responsibility for any possible consequences from any treatment, procedure, exercise, dietary modification, action or application of medication which results from reading or following the information contained in this information. The publication of this information does not constitute the practice of medicine, and this information does not replace the advice of your physician or other health care provider.

The Natural Path to Hormonal Wellness, Part 1 by Katarina Nolte
Pages: 201 (23,609 words); Copyright © 2014 by Katarina Nolte.
All rights reserved. http://katarinanolte.com/ July 2014

BLURB

Are you suffering from hormonal imbalance?
Do you feel stressed, tired and out of energy?
Are you worried about environmental estrogens?
Are you looking for natural ways to detoxify and regenerate your mind-body system?
Are you interested in taking charge of your hormonal balance?
Do you see yourself making your own herbal preparations and meals containing hormone balancing nutrients?
Have you ever wondered what our ancestors were consuming to support overall wellness, libido and longevity?

If the above applies to you, read **"The Natural Path to Hormonal Wellness, Part 1"** and get started!

The Natural Path to Hormonal Wellness, Part 1 by Katarina Nolte
Pages: 201 (23,609 words); Copyright © 2014 by Katarina Nolte.
All rights reserved. http://katarinanolte.com/ July 2014

ACKNOWLEDGEMENTS

I would like to express my gratitude to all the people who publish and otherwise share practical information on the subject of wellness.

The Natural Path to Hormonal Wellness, Part 1 by Katarina Nolte
Pages: 201 (23,609 words); Copyright © 2014 by Katarina Nolte.
All rights reserved. http://katarinanolte.com/ July 2014

INTRODUCTION

Three of the most common health issues affecting people today are fat gain, digestive issues and hormonal imbalances, all of which are diseases of civilization and each of which can be the cause of the other.

Digestive issues can lead to hormonal imbalances and hormonal imbalances can lead to digestive issues. Fat gain can lead to hormonal imbalances and hormonal imbalances can lead to fat gain. Digestive issues can lead to fat gain and fat gain can lead to digestive issues.

Pollution, chronic stress, excessive sugar consumption, industrial food, and our typically sedentary lifestyle limited to the indoors, all wreck havoc on the delicate mind-body balance known as homeostasis. A vital part of homeostasis is hormonal balance.

In my new book series "The Natural Path to Hormonal Wellness", I am exploring the natural ways to regain this important internal balance. My goal is to create detailed lists of hormone balancing herbs, antioxidants, amino acids, foods, and more, beginning with "The Natural Path to Hormonal Wellness, Part 1".

As the title indicates, the focus is on wellness. The herbs and other nutrients I begin the series with are all used for multiple purposes. This means that these natural substances are not magic pills and yet they have been used for ages to support and strengthen the mind-body system as a whole.

LEARN

1. How to make 15 different herbal preparations;
2. Where the most popular 23 hormone balancing herbs come from;
3. What they are used for traditionally and otherwise;
4. Which types of nutrients they contain;
5. Their commercial availability;
6. The most effective ways to consume them;
7. 5 additional hormone balancing nutrients and their uses and sources.

The Natural Path to Hormonal Wellness, Part 1 by Katarina Nolte
Pages: 201 (23,609 words); Copyright © 2014 by Katarina Nolte.
All rights reserved. http://katarinanolte.com/ July 2014

ESTROGEN DOMINANCE SYMPTOMS

Strictly speaking, it's possible that we are all -- men, women and children -- suffering a little from estrogen dominance, because there is so much of it in our environment. You would have to virtually live in a bubble to escape the excess estrogens we're exposed to through pesticides, plastics, industrial waste products, car exhaust, meat, soaps and much of the carpeting, furniture and paneling that we live with indoors every day.
Estrogen Dominance | JohnLeeMD
http://www.johnleemd.com/store/estrogen_dom.html

1. Fat gain
2. Low energy
3. Sexual/reproductive dysfunction
4. Aches and pains
5. Chronic conditions
6. Female problems in puberty, adulthood, premenopause, perimenopause, and menopause
7. Developmental problems and premature aging
8. Inability to maintain homeostasis
9. Depression, addiction
10. Cancer

LEARN MORE

Estrogens, xenoestrogens, dominance, treatment | Grow Youthful
http://www.growyouthful.com/ailment/estrogen.php

Xenoestrogens and The Brain | Center For Brain Training
http://www.centerforbrain.com/xenoestrogens-and-the-brain/

Progesterone Dominance | Natural-Hormones.net
http://www.natural-hormones.net/progesterone-dominance.htm

Rhythmic Living » Symptoms of Progesterone Toxicity
http://rhythmicliving.org/?page_id=60

Rhythmic Living » Progesterone Detox
http://rhythmicliving.org/?page_id=123

The Natural Path to Hormonal Wellness, Part 1 by Katarina Nolte
Pages: 201 (23,609 words); Copyright © 2014 by Katarina Nolte.
All rights reserved. http://katarinanolte.com/ July 2014

HORMONAL TIDBITS

*One of the concerning discoveries of the study was
the observation that the decline in fertility for
women 15-24 of age was very similar to the decline
for women aged 25 years and over.*
**Crowded Waiting Rooms: It's Time for Women to
Wake-Up to What's Beneath Rising Infertility Rates
| The Shift Network**
http://theshiftnetwork.com/blog/2014-01-
25/crowded-waiting-rooms-its-time-women-wake-
whats-beneath-rising-infertility-rates

Standard hormone tests do not test for the
presence of artificial estrogens. Artificial estrogens
are similar but not identical to the body's own
estrogens and are more damaging. We ingest them
via air, water, food and industrial products.

Very many, if not most, manmade chemicals are
xenoestrogenic. Identifying them in one's system
would require one blood, urine, and/or hair test for
each and every manmade chemical in existence.
That would be exorbitantly expensive and time
consuming.

This also means that people whose mind-body
systems are suffering from estrogen overload are
not diagnosed as being estrogen dominant.
Further, estrogen dominance in its true sense
means that there is an excess of total estrogens in
proportion to most other hormones, including but
not limited to testosterone and progesterone.

The Natural Path to Hormonal Wellness, Part 1 by Katarina Nolte
Pages: 201 (23,609 words); Copyright © 2014 by Katarina Nolte.
All rights reserved. http://katarinanolte.com/ July 2014

Bioidentical progesterone is often promoted as the solution to excessive levels of estrogens. What is rarely mentioned is that the symptoms of progesterone dominance resemble the symptoms of estrogen dominance. And the symptoms of progesterone deficiency resemble those of progesterone dominance.

Estrogen dominance symptoms resemble the symptoms of (endogenous) estrogen insufficiency. The symptoms of estrogen dominance also resemble the symptoms of testosterone deficiency in female, male, younger and older adults.

Excess testosterone inadvertently leads to excess estrogen at which point the symptoms of excess estrogen are incorrectly attributed to excess testosterone. A state of excess testosterone/testosterone dominance is, by the way, pretty much impossible as any excesses either aromatize into estrogen or convert into dihydrotestosterone (DHT), or are swiftly flushed out of the system.

DHT, like estrogen, is associated with hair loss and prostate issues. It is increasingly suspected that DHT may be closer related to estrogen than to testosterone.

The Natural Path to Hormonal Wellness, Part 1 by Katarina Nolte
Pages: 201 (23,609 words); Copyright © 2014 by Katarina Nolte.
All rights reserved. http://katarinanolte.com/ July 2014

The question of androgen deficiency has largely been ignored in pre-menopausal women... In reality, women may develop symptoms of androgen deficiency at any age, from their teen years through late adulthood.

Androgen deficiency in women | Better Health Channel

http://www.betterhealth.vic.gov.au/bhcv2/bhcarticles.nsf/pages/Androgen_deficiency_in_women

TESTOSTERONE DEFICIENCY SYMPTOMS

The reality is that testosterone deficiency is an extremely common condition affecting men and women of all adult age groups. It robs us of our strength, energy, and sexuality. It damages our psyche and affects our personal relationships. It is a cause of, or a great contributor to, a wide range of diseases that result in illness, debility, and, ultimately, death.

Testosterone Deficiency | The Hidden Disease by E. Barry Gordon, M.D.

http://www.thehiddendisease.com/tdthedisease.html

1. See ESTROGEN DOMINACE SYMPTOMS
2. Low drive/self-esteem
3. Connective tissue weakness
4. Diminished brain function
5. Irritability, anxiety
6. Autoimmune disease
7. Cardiovascular issues
8. Respiratory issues
9. Gastrointestinal issues

As we can see, hormones and hormonal imbalances affect the entire mind-body system. One of the simplest ways to try to regain homeostasis is to avoid toxins and rearrange our diet and lifestyle with the goal to remove toxins on a consistent and permanent basis. And when it comes to results, it is best to focus on overall

The Natural Path to Hormonal Wellness, Part 1 by Katarina Nolte
Pages: 201 (23,609 words); Copyright © 2014 by Katarina Nolte.
All rights reserved. http://katarinanolte.com/ July 2014

wellbeing, because wellness and fitness are attained in little steps.

On average phytoestrogens are about 200 to 400 times weaker than the body's own estrogen. So they have a duel effect by both acting as very weak estrogens and by locking up estrogen receptors to block the action of stronger and more dangerous estrogens. For instance Premarin (PREgnant MARes urINe), which is 3,000 times stronger than human estrogen, and xenoestrogens, such as dioxin and PCBs, which can be as high as 30,000 times stronger than human estrogens.

Progesterone dominance and hormone balance at The Truth in Medicine, message 1521544 | Cure Zone

http://curezone.org/forums/fm.asp?i=1521544

The Natural Path to Hormonal Wellness, Part 1 by Katarina Nolte
Pages: 201 (23,609 words); Copyright © 2014 by Katarina Nolte.
All rights reserved. http://katarinanolte.com/ July 2014

HOW TO MAKE HERBAL PREPARATIONS

The biological or therapeutic activity of a medicinal plant is closely related to the plant chemicals in it. These chemicals can be classified into major groups of chemicals such as essential oils, alkaloids, acids, steroids, tannins, saponins and so forth. Each one of these classes of chemicals may have a preferred effective method of extraction which facilitates getting the chemicals out of the plant and into the herbal remedy that is being prepared. For example, some active chemicals found in plants are not soluble or dissolved in water, therefore just preparing a hot tea with the plant, or even boiling the plant in hot water won't extract these chemicals into the resulting water extract/tea remedy. Generally, if they aren't water soluble, they won't be broken down in the digestive process either, so taking the plant in capsules or tablets won't be much help either.
Herbal Preparation Methods | Rain Tree
http://www.rain-tree.com/prepmethod.htm#.U3196dJdWSo

TEA

1. Pour filtered water into a ceramic tea kettle and bring to a boil.
2. Pour the boiled water into a ceramic or glass cup.
3. Add your herb/s. If it's a powder, add one or two teaspoonfuls. Use a wooden, glass or ceramic spoon to do this. Do not use metal with your herbs. If it's not a powder, you can use a cotton teabag.
4. Cover with a fitting ceramic, wooden or glass plate and let sit for 15 minutes or more.
5. Ideally, consume pure with no additional ingredients and do so within 24 hours.

LEARN MORE

Are Glazed Ceramic Pans and Cookware Safe? - Wellness Mama
http://wellnessmama.com/13203/glazed-ceramic-pans-safe/
Joyce Chen Ceramic Tea Kettle with Bamboo Handle - Park and Main
http://www.parkandmain.com/products/Joyce-Chen-Ceramic-Tea-Kettle-with-Bamboo-Handle.html
Amazon.com: Bamboo Wood Cooking Spoon - 12 Inch: Wooden Spoons: Kitchen & Dining
http://www.amazon.com/Bamboo-Wood-Cooking-Spoon-Inch/dp/B004IFTS9C

The Natural Path to Hormonal Wellness, Part 1 by Katarina Nolte
Pages: 201 (23,609 words); Copyright © 2014 by Katarina Nolte.
All rights reserved. http://katarinanolte.com/ July 2014

HOT INFUSION

1. Pour filtered water into a ceramic tea kettle and bring to a boil.
2. Pour the boiled water into a ceramic or glass jar with a sealable ceramic or glass lid and without metal coming into direct contact with the infusion.
3. Add your herb/s. If it's a powder, add one or two teaspoonfuls per teacup. Use a wooden, glass or ceramic spoon to do this. Do not use metal with your herbs. If it's not a powder, you can use a cotton teabag.
4. Lock tightly and let sit for 4-10 hours.
5. Ideally, consume pure with no additional ingredients and do so within 24 hours.

LEARN MORE

Amazon.com: Le Parfait French Glass Canning Jar with 85mm Gasket and Lid - 3/4 (.75) Liter: Kitchen & Dining
http://www.amazon.com/Parfait-French-Glass-Canning-Gasket/dp/B001A5QQ52

COLD INFUSION

1. Fill a ceramic or glass jar with a sealable ceramic or glass lid with your herbs.
2. Pour unheated filtered water over them and lock tightly.
3. Let sit for 48 hours away from direct light.
4. Strain thoroughly into a ceramic or glass container with a sealable ceramic or glass lid using a cheesecloth.
5. Ideally, consume pure with no additional ingredients and do so within 24 hours.

Don't use city tap water that contains chlorine, use either distilled or pure spring water.
Tinctures And Herbal Extracts: How To Make | Annie's Remedy
http://www.anniesremedy.com/chart_remedy_extracts.php

The Natural Path to Hormonal Wellness, Part 1 by Katarina Nolte
Pages: 201 (23,609 words); Copyright © 2014 by Katarina Nolte.
All rights reserved. http://katarinanolte.com/ July 2014

INFUSED OIL

1. Fill a ceramic or glass jar with a sealable ceramic or glass lid with your herbs.
2. Pour your choice of edible, cold pressed, unrefined oils (olive, grape seed, avocado, sesame, etc.) over them and lock tightly.
3. Let sit for 4 days in a warm, dark and dry location.
4. Strain thoroughly into a ceramic or glass container with a sealable ceramic or glass lid using a cheesecloth.
5. Ideally, consume pure with no additional ingredients (externally or internally) and do so within 3 months.

NOTE

Store in a ceramic or glass jar with a sealable ceramic or glass lid in a dry, dark place and do not expose to direct light or varying temperatures.

LEARN MORE

Herb Pharm │Infused Herbal Oils & Essential Oils, What's the Difference?
http://www.herb-pharm.com/Herb_Pharm_oils_article.html
How to Make Herbal Infused Oils ‑ YouTube
http://youtu.be/e095va7iAX0

The Natural Path to Hormonal Wellness, Part 1 by Katarina Nolte
Pages: 201 (23,609 words); Copyright © 2014 by Katarina Nolte.
All rights reserved. http://katarinanolte.com/ July 2014

How to Make a Herbal Infused Oil | Whispering Earth

http://whisperingearth.co.uk/2010/04/26/potions-group-making-herb-infused-oils/

The Natural Path to Hormonal Wellness, Part 1 by Katarina Nolte
Pages: 201 (23,609 words); Copyright © 2014 by Katarina Nolte.
All rights reserved. http://katarinanolte.com/ July 2014

DECOCTION

1. Place your herbs into a ceramic tea kettle (1-2 wooden, ceramic or glass teaspoons per teacup).
2. Add filtered water.
3. Adjust the heat to medium to medium-high and bring to a boil.
4. Reduce heat to a simmer (low to medium-low) and simmer for 20-60 minutes.
5. Let cool to warm to lukewarm.
6. Strain thoroughly using a cheesecloth into a glass or ceramic container with a sealable ceramic or glass lid.
7. Ideally, consume pure with no additional ingredients (externally or internally) and do so within 72 hours.

NOTE

For increased potency, presoak the herbs in unheated, filtered water overnight in a ceramic or glass jar with a sealable ceramic or glass lid located in a dry, dark place and do not expose to direct light or varying temperatures. Then, proceed with step one.

LEARN MORE

Herbal Decoctions: Remedies, Recipes, How To Make │Annie's Remedy
http://www.anniesremedy.com/chart_remedy_decoction.php

Explaining Herbal Decoctions-One Method in Using Herbs - Yahoo Voices
http://voices.yahoo.com/explaining-herbal-decoctions-one-method-using-herbs-7501020.html
Decoction - Wikipedia, the free encyclopedia
http://en.wikipedia.org/wiki/Decoction
What is the difference between a decoction and an infusion │Health Freedom
http://www.healthfreedom.info/Decoction%20v.%20Infusion.htm
Amazon.com: Pyrex Prepware 2-Cup Measuring Cup, Clear with Red Measurements: Kitchen & Dining
http://www.amazon.com/Pyrex-Prepware-2-Cup-Measuring-Measurements/dp/B0002ITQHS/
Glass Bottles – Mountain Rose Herbs
https://www.mountainroseherbs.com/catalog/glass-bottles

The Natural Path to Hormonal Wellness, Part 1 by Katarina Nolte
Pages: 201 (23,609 words); Copyright © 2014 by Katarina Nolte.
All rights reserved. http://katarinanolte.com/ July 2014

TINCTURE

1. Fill a ceramic or glass jar with a sealable ceramic or glass lid with your herbs.
2. Pour a choice of drinkable alcohol like vodka, rum or brandy (preferably organic) over them and lock tightly.
3. Let sit for 2-6 weeks in a cool, dry and dark location
4. Gently shake the container once or twice daily during the period.
5. Strain thoroughly into a ceramic or glass container with a sealable ceramic or glass lid using a cheesecloth.
6. Ideally, consume pure with no additional ingredients (internally or externally) and do so within 6 months.
7. Store in a in a cool, dry and dark location.

NOTE

If your herbs are ground or crushed, use 2 ounces for each pint of alcohol.

NOTE 2

Alcohol, like sugar, is counter effective. Both are known to lead to hormonal imbalance.

LEARN MORE

How to Make an Herbal Tincture » Meridian Massage Institute
http://meridianmassageinstitute.com/remedies/how-to-make-an-herbal-tincture/

Combination Herbal Extracts – Mountain Rose Herbs
https://www.mountainroseherbs.com/catalog/extracts/combinations

How to Make Your Own Herbal Tinctures │Nature's Apotheke
http://www.naturesapotheke.com/howtomakeyourownherbaltinctures.htm

Schramm Organic Potato Vodka │Pembert on Distillery
http://www.pembertondistillery.ca/vodka.html

Gluten-Free Vodka List │Celiac Disease │About.com
http://celiacdisease.about.com/od/GlutenFreeAlcohol/a/Gluten-Free-Vodka-List.htm

American Harvest Organic Spirit
http://americanharvestspirit.com/

Why Muslin is the Better Cheesecloth - Viet World Kitchen
http://www.vietworldkitchen.com/blog/2012/03/muslin-is-the-better-cheesecloth.html

Amazon.com: Regency Natural Ultra Fine 100% Cotton Cheesecloth 9sq.ft: Kitchen & Dining
http://www.amazon.com/Regency-Natural-Cotton-Cheesecloth-9sq-ft/dp/B001B14ODG

How to make Herbal Preparations│Dr Standley
http://www.drstandley.com/supplements_herbal_preparations.shtml

Guide to Making Tinctures « The Mountain Rose Blog
http://mountainroseblog.com/guide-tinctures-extracts/

Books on Herbal Medicine – Mountain Rose Herbs

https://www.mountainroseherbs.com/catalog/education/herbal-medicine

ALCOHOL OR GLYCERIN BASED HERBAL EXTRACT

1. Fill a ceramic or glass jar with a sealable ceramic or glass lid with your herbs.
2. Add a choice of drinkable alcohol like vodka, rum or brandy (preferably organic) over them at a proportion of 20% herb 80% alcohol and lock tightly. Organic glycerin can be used instead.
3. Lock tightly and let sit for 4-6 weeks in a cool, dry and dark location.
4. Gently shake the container once a day during the period.
5. Strain thoroughly into a ceramic or glass container with a sealable ceramic or glass lid using a cheesecloth.
6. Ideally, consume pure with no additional ingredients (internally or externally) and do so within 6 months.
7. Store in a in a cool, dry and dark location.

NOTE

Alcohol, like sugar, is counter effective. Both are known to lead to hormonal imbalance.

LEARN MORE

Make Your Own Liquid Herbal Extract - Mountain Rose Herbs
https://www.mountainroseherbs.com/learn/herbal-extracts

**Can I make extracts without alcohol? | Yahoo
Answers**

https://answers.yahoo.com/question/index?qid=20100
327162045AAbGr1W

Vegetable Glycerine – Mountain Rose Herbs

https://www.mountainroseherbs.com/products/vegeta
ble-glycerine/profile

The Natural Path to Hormonal Wellness, Part 1 by Katarina Nolte
Pages: 201 (23,609 words); Copyright © 2014 by Katarina Nolte.
All rights reserved. http://katarinanolte.com/ July 2014

INFUSED VINEGAR/HERBAL VINEGAR EXTRACT

1. Fill a quarter of a ceramic or glass jar with a sealable ceramic or glass lid with your herbs.
2. Fill the rest of the jar with raw, organic apple cider vinegar with mother.
3. Lock tightly and let sit for two weeks in a cool, dry and dark location.
4. Gently shake once or twice a day during the period.
5. Strain thoroughly into a ceramic or glass container with a sealable ceramic or glass lid using a cheesecloth.
6. Ideally, consume pure with no additional ingredients (internally or externally) and do so within 6 months.
7. Store in a in a cool, dry and dark location.

LEARN MORE

The Benefits of Apple Cider Vinegar - Global Healing Center
http://www.globalhealingcenter.com/natural-health/the-benefits-of-apple-cider-vinegar/
8 Amazing Uses for Apple Cider Vinegar │Gerson Institute
http://gerson.org/gerpress/8-amazing-uses-for-apple-cider-vinegar/
How to Make Medicinal Vinegar « The Mountain Rose Blog
http://mountainroseblog.com/medicinal-vinegars/
How to Make Essential Oils: 16 Steps (with Pictures) - wikiHow
http://www.wikihow.com/Make-Essential-Oils

The Natural Path to Hormonal Wellness, Part 1 by Katarina Nolte
Pages: 201 (23,609 words); Copyright © 2014 by Katarina Nolte.
All rights reserved. http://katarinanolte.com/ July 2014

How to Make Flower Essence Remedies -Herbal Medicine - YouTube

http://www.youtube.com/watch?v=q6NYNgcfXNU

The Natural Path to Hormonal Wellness, Part 1 by Katarina Nolte
Pages: 201 (23,609 words); Copyright © 2014 by Katarina Nolte.
All rights reserved. http://katarinanolte.com/ July 2014

OINTMENT

1. Fill the lower part of a Pyrex double boiler with water and bring to a simmering boil.
2. Pour 8 ounces of your choice of edible, cold pressed, unrefined oils (olive, grape seed, avocado, sesame, etc.) into the upper part of the Pyrex double boiler.
3. Reduce the heat to low to medium low.
4. Add an ounce of organic beeswax to the oil.
5. Once the beeswax has melted, remove from the stove and pour into a glass or ceramic bowl.
6. Add a dozen or so drops of one or more herbal tinctures, extracts and/or essential oils and stir gently.
7. Cover with a fitting ceramic or glass plate and let sit for 30 minutes or until cool.
8. Store in a ceramic or glass jar with a sealable ceramic or glass lid in the refrigerator.

NOTE

Cacao butter or shea butter can also be added to the oils.

NOTE 2

External use only.

The Natural Path to Hormonal Wellness, Part 1 by Katarina Nolte
Pages: 201 (23,609 words); Copyright © 2014 by Katarina Nolte.
All rights reserved. http://katarinanolte.com/ July 2014

LEARN MORE

Ingredients for preparing ointments and creams |Heil Kraeuter

http://en.heilkraeuter.net/ointment/ingredients.htm

HERBAL SALVE

1. Fill the lower part of a Pyrex double boiler with water and bring to a simmering boil.
2. Reduce temperature to low to medium low.
3. Pour a total of 8 ounces of one or more infused oils into the upper part of the Pyrex double boiler.
4. Place one ounce of organic beeswax into the oil until the beeswax is fully melted.
5. Remove from the stove and pour into a ceramic or glass jar with a sealable ceramic or glass lid.
6. Stir gently a few times with a wooden spatula and lock tightly.
7. Allow for it to cool completely at room temperature.
8. Store in the refrigerator and use within a year.

NOTE

You can add additional herbal tinctures and/or essential oils prior to cooling.

NOTE 2

External use only.

LEARN MORE

How to Make Herbal Salve - YouTube
http://youtu.be/RqDq_VnZ8Ok
Waxes – Mountain Rose Herbs
https://www.mountainroseherbs.com/catalog/waxes

Amazon.com: 100% ORGANIC Hand Poured Beeswax - ~1oz each - Premium Quality, Cosmetic Grade, Triple Filtered Bees Wax (5 or 6 Bars; Additional Bar May Be Included to Make Sure Minimum of 5oz of Beeswax): Health & Personal Care
http://www.amazon.com/100-ORGANIC-Hand-Poured-Beeswax/dp/B00455IWK6

Amber Brown Pyrex Sauce Pan from the Corning Ware by DeAnnasAttic │Etsy
https://www.etsy.com/listing/166225005/amber-brown-pyrex-sauce-pan-from-the

What Happened to the Glass Double Boiler? │ Holy Scrap Hot Springs Blog
http://blog.holyscraphotsprings.com/2010/06/what-happened-to-glass-double-boiler.html

DIY: Herbal Salves « The Mountain Rose Blog
http://mountainroseblog.com/diy-herbal-salves/

Herbal Salves │ Frontier Natural Products Co-op
http://www.frontiercoop.com/learn/herbalsalves.php

HERBAL SKIN CREAM

1. Fill the lower part of a Pyrex double boiler with water and bring to a simmering boil.
2. Reduce temperature to low to medium low.
3. Pour a total of 8 ounces of one or more infused oils into the upper part of the Pyrex double boiler.
4. Place one ounce of organic beeswax into the oil until the beeswax is fully melted.
5. Remove from the stove and pour into a ceramic or glass bowl and let cool to lukewarm.
6. Add several drops of one or more herbal tinctures and/or essential oils.
7. Start mixing the liquid using a hand mixer.
8. Simultaneously, begin adding tiny amounts of an 8-ounce herbal decoction.
9. Once the desired thickness has been achieved, turn off the mixer and begin transferring the cream into a ceramic or glass jar with a sealable ceramic or glass lid using a wooden, glass or ceramic spoon or spatula.
10. Store in the refrigerator and use within 3 months.

NOTE

For external use only.

LEARN MORE

How To Make A Cream - Herbalism Basics 6 - YouTube
http://youtu.be/2gkDoMNz8RQ

Fido .5-Liter Jar with Clamp Lid in Outlet Kitchen | Crate and Barrel

http://www.crateandbarrel.com/fido-.5-liter-jar-with-clamp-lid/s495053

Fido 1-Liter Jar with Clamp Lid in Outlet Kitchen | Crate and Barrel

http://www.crateandbarrel.com/fido-1-liter-jar-with-clamp-lid/s495118

Herbalism - YouTube

http://www.youtube.com/playlist?list=PLF15749FA23620164

The Natural Path to Hormonal Wellness, Part 1 by Katarina Nolte
Pages: 201 (23,609 words); Copyright © 2014 by Katarina Nolte.
All rights reserved. http://katarinanolte.com/ July 2014

SOAKS AND BATHS

1. Fill the tub or a ceramic bowl with comfortably warm water.
2. Add your choice of an herbal preparation or fresh or dried herbs.
3. Soak your feet/body for 10 minutes.

NOTE

Do not immerse any metal or plastic items like manicure or pedicure tools in your herbal bath water.

The Natural Path to Hormonal Wellness, Part 1 by Katarina Nolte
Pages: 201 (23,609 words); Copyright © 2014 by Katarina Nolte.

FACIAL STEAMING

1. Pour filtered water into a ceramic tea kettle and bring to a boil.
2. Pour the boiled water into a ceramic or glass bowl.
3. Add your choice of an herbal preparation or fresh or dried herbs.
4. Cover with a plate and let sit for 10-15 minutes.
5. Place the bowl on the dining table and sit with your face over it and your head covered with a towel.
6. Inhale, raise the towel and exhale. Repeat a dozen or so times.

NOTE

Do not apply any metal or plastic items like cosmetology tools to your skin. Rinse off the herbal preparation first.

COMPRESS

1. Pour filtered water into a ceramic tea kettle and bring to a boil.
2. Pour the boiled water into a ceramic or glass container.
3. Add your choice of herb/s as if making a tea.
4. Cover with a fitting ceramic, wooden or glass plate and let sit for 5 minutes.
5. Immerse a cheesecloth into the liquid.
6. Squeeze out excess liquid and apply to the affected area.
7. Once the poultice has cooled, repeat the process for as long the tea is warm enough to be effective.

NOTE

Don't allow direct contact between your herbal preparation and metal.

NOTE 2

You can add a few drops of an herbal tincture of choice to the tea or the cheesecloth for added effect.

HERBAL PASTE POULTICE

1. Pour filtered water into a ceramic tea kettle and bring to a boil.
2. Pour a tiny amount of the boiled water into a small ceramic or stone bowl. Mortar and pestle are best for this.
3. Add your choice of herb/s. Ideally, use crushed or ground herbs.
4. Apply pressure using the pestle until you get a pasty consistency.
5. Moisten a cheesecloth in an herbal tea preparation or a liquid consisting of warm water and a few drops of an herbal tincture (or extract).
6. Spread the cheesecloth onto a plate and fill it with your herbal paste as if making a roll.
7. Place on the affected area.

LEARN MORE

The Difference between Tinctures, Tonics and Teas... Oh My! | Nourishing Herbalist
http://www.nourishingherbalist.com/the-difference-between-tinctures-tonics-and-teas-oh-my/
Mortar and pestle - Wikipedia, the free encyclopedia
http://en.wikipedia.org/wiki/Mortar_and_pestle
Herbal Poultices | Frontier Natural Products Co-op
https://www.frontiercoop.com/learn/herbalpoultices.php

The Natural Path to Hormonal Wellness, Part 1 by Katarina Nolte
Pages: 201 (23,609 words); Copyright © 2014 by Katarina Nolte.
All rights reserved. http://katarinanolte.com/ July 2014

HERBAL PREPARATION RULES AND SUGGESTIONS

Maintain proper hygiene and sanitation.

Do not bring herb and herbal preparations into direct contact with metal and preferably avoid plastic as well.

Use ceramic, Pyrex glass, stone and wooden tools for the preparation and storage.

Try to obtain organic, unpolluted, fresh and eco-friendly herbs and tools.

Keep in mind that some herbs are known by more than one name, while others have similar sounding names. Whenever possible, check the Latin name of each herb you are interested in obtaining.

Ideally purchase bulk herbs online from companies who specialize in herbs. This choice also happens to be the most economical one.

Use filtered water and organic, edible oils in your herbal preparations.

If your goal is to benefit from herbal phytosterols specifically, keep in mind that these may be altered and/or destroyed by alcohol, high heat and/or vinegar.

The most benefit from the consumption of herbs can be gained by them being prepared traditionally. That is, the way a given herb has been prepared and consumed since the folk tradition has been established.

LEARN MORE

How to Make Your Own Herbal Preparations | Herba Luna
http://www.herbaluna.com/How-To-Make-Your-Own-Herbal-Preparations.php
Different Kinds Of Herbal Preparations Explained | Herb Geek
http://www.herbgeek.com/different-kinds-of-herbal-preparations-explained/
Wild Health: Lessons in Natural Wellness from the Animal Kingdom - Cindy Engel - Google Books
http://books.google.com/books/about/Wild_Health.html?id=8FwqLh2a2ckC
Making Herbal Preparations | Wicca
http://wicca.com/celtic/herbal/herbalpreps.htm
Henriette's Herbal Homepage
http://www.henriettes-herb.com/
Methow Valley Herbs: What's Chemistry Got to do With It?
http://www.methowvalleyherbs.com/2008/09/whats-chemistry-got-to-do-with-it.html

Avoid using pots made of steel, iron, and any other metal. Some herbs react to them.
How to Make an Herbal Tincture: 8 Steps (with Pictures) - wikiHow
http://www.wikihow.com/Make-an-Herbal-Tincture

The Natural Path to Hormonal Wellness, Part 1 by Katarina Nolte
Pages: 201 (23,609 words); Copyright © 2014 by Katarina Nolte.
All rights reserved. http://katarinanolte.com/ July 2014

HERBS

ASTRAGALUS

From an herbal standpoint, Mindy recommends Siberian ginseng, as opposed to regular ginseng, and astragalus, which is also good for immune support, as key tonics for the adrenal and endocrine systems. In their book Herbal Defense, herbalists Robyn Landis and K.P. Khalsa discusses the benefits of Siberian Ginseng and astragalus.
Adrenal Fatigue / Adrenal Exhaustion and the Thyroid | Thyroid | About.com
http://thyroid.about.com/cs/endocrinology/a/adrenalfatigue_2.htm

Astragalus (Astragalus membranaceus) is a plant belonging to the bean and pea family (legumes). There are thousands of Astragalus species, dozens of which have been used medicinally since ancient times in Asia (China, Mongolia, Korea, Iranian Plateau, and India).

Astragalus is an adaptogen and as such it helps the mind-body system regain homeostasis. If successful, it may lead to hormonal balance and more bioavailable testosterone, among other mild improvements in overall wellbeing.

Astragalus should be cycled — 3 weeks on and 1
week off, or 2 weeks on 2 weeks off — or used
irregularly (1-2 times/week).

ASTRAGALUS USES

- Immune system support
- Longevity, antiaging, regeneration, and
rejuvenation
- Cardiovascular health
- Respiratory health
- Detoxification (liver, kidney, lymph tissues)
- Chronic disease prevention and treatment
- Edema prevention
- Vitality, energy, spirit, and stamina
- Sexual and reproductive function
- Rest and recovery support, athletic and otherwise
- Gastrointestinal health
- Pain alleviation
- Blood sugar balance
- Stress management (adrenal health)
- Anti-inflammatory, anti-cancer, anti-tumor,
antioxidant, antibacterial, antiviral

In addition to its adaptogenic properties,
astragalus is also an herbal energy tonic and has
been used as a protective measure following
radiation exposure.

The medicinal astragalus root contains saponins,
polysaccharides, beta-sitosterol, flavonoids,
betaine, essential fatty acids, choline, magnesium,
calcium, zinc, manganese, iron, and selenium.

Astragalus is consumed as a tea, capsule, extract, decoction, tincture, and powder.

Traditional preparation: tea, extract.

NOTE

Do not consume with sugar or sweeteners. Sugar and sweeteners are counter effective to hormonal balance.

LEARN MORE

Astragalus "super herb" protects, supports immune system function | Natural News
http://www.naturalnews.com/027223_ASTRAGALUS_i
mmune_system.html#
Astragalus - Wikipedia, the free encyclopedia
http://en.wikipedia.org/wiki/Astragalus#Traditional_u
ses
Astragalus Extract - Mountain Rose Herbs
https://www.mountainroseherbs.com/products/astrag
alus-extract/profile
The spleen is a type of blood cell filter | Hannen Health
http://hannenhealth.com/spleen.htm
Healing Glands and Organs 101: The Liver and Spleen
http://healingyou101-
glandsandorgans.blogspot.com/2008/12/liver-and-
spleen.html
Lymph Drainage for Detoxification | Massage Therapy Articles
http://www.massagetherapy.com/articles/index.php/a
rticle_id/1200/Lymph-Drainage-for-Detoxification-

The Natural Path to Hormonal Wellness, Part 1 by Katarina Nolte
Pages: 201 (23,609 words); Copyright © 2014 by Katarina Nolte.
All rights reserved. http://katarinanolte.com/ July 2014

11 Ways to Boost Your Lymphatic System for Great Health | Care2 Healthy Living
http://www.care2.com/greenliving/11-ways-to-boost-your-lymphatic-system-for-great-health.html

How to Grow Astragalus | Guide to Growing Astragalus
http://www.heirloom-organics.com/guide/va/guidetogrowingastragalus.html

How to Grow Astragalus at Home | Buzzle
http://www.buzzle.com/articles/how-to-grow-astragalus-at-home.html

Crop rotation for herbs│GrowFruitAndVeg.co.uk
http://www.growfruitandveg.co.uk/grapevine/new-shoots/crop-rotation-herbs_2118.html

Methow Valley Herbs: Astragalus: A Supreme Protector
http://www.methowvalleyherbs.com/2012/02/astragalus-supreme-protector.html

Astragalus Health Benefits: It Stops Aging, Cancer, And More! │ Health Kismet Blog
http://blog.healthkismet.com/astragalus-health-benefits

Astragalus │ Healthelicious
http://www.healthelicious.com.au/ingredients/Astragalus.html

Radix Astragalus and testosterone - Paleohacks
http://paleohacks.com/questions/65707/radix-astragalus-and-testosterone.html

The Natural Path to Hormonal Wellness, Part 1 by Katarina Nolte
Pages: 201 (23,609 words); Copyright © 2014 by Katarina Nolte.
All rights reserved. http://katarinanolte.com/ July 2014

6. Rotate the use of herbs. Generally, use herbs six days on and one day off. For example, use herbs Mon - Sat., and take Sundays off. Use herbs as recommended or, as a general rule, for 6-12 weeks, then rotate off one whole week to allow your body's own healing mechanisms to take over. Resume your program the following week. Use a calendar to keep track.

Get the Most Out of Your Healing Regime - Learn the Best Way to Take Herbs and Supplements - Yahoo Voices - voices.yahoo.com

http://voices.yahoo.com/get-most-out-healing-regime-learn-the-305393.html

ASHWAGANDHA

Most people aren't aware that you can start with an excellent high-quality properly grown herb, but if it is not harvested at the correct time and then optimally processed a great deal of the herbal potency can be lost... And that's why I do not recommend you pick up any ashwagandha (or any herb) from your local grocery store. I've seen far too many herbs containing artificial ingredients and ones that use questionable chemical processes. You're better off not taking the herb at all if this is the case.

Ashwagandha | Organic Herbal Supplements - Mercola.com

http://organicindia.mercola.com/herbal-supplements/ashwagandha.aspx

Ashwagandha (Withania somnifera) is an ancient Ayurvedic (Indian) herb also found in Western Asia and North Africa.

Ashwagandha is an adaptogen and as such it helps the mind-body system regain homeostasis. If successful, it may lead to hormonal balance and more bioavailable testosterone, among other mild improvements in overall wellbeing.

Ashwagandha should be cycled — 3 weeks on and 1 week off, or 2 weeks on 2 weeks off — or used irregularly (1-2 times/week).

ASHWAGANDHA USES

- Stress management (adrenal/thyroid health)
- Neuroprotective and neuroregenerative
- Connective tissue strengthening
- Longevity, antiaging, regeneration, and rejuvenation
- Detoxification (liver, kidney, lymph tissues)
- Vitality, energy, spirit, and stamina
- Sexual and reproductive function
- Rest and recovery support, athletic and otherwise
- Blood sugar balance
- Pain alleviation
- Immune system support
- Gastrointestinal health
- Anti-inflammatory, antioxidant, anti-cancer, anti-tumor, antifungal, and antibacterial

The medicinal Ashwagandha roots and berries contain beta-sitosterol, amino acids, and choline.

Ashwagandha can be consumed raw, whole, dried and ground (powder), as a capsule, tea, or tincture.

Traditional preparation: root decoction.

NOTE

Do not consume with sugar or sweeteners. Sugar and sweeteners are counter effective to hormonal balance.

The Natural Path to Hormonal Wellness, Part 1 by Katarina Nolte
Pages: 201 (23,609 words); Copyright © 2014 by Katarina Nolte.
All rights reserved. http://katarinanolte.com/ July 2014

LEARN MORE

Ashwagandha: Stress Reduction, Neural Protection, and a Lot More from an Ancient Herb - Life Extension
https://www.lef.org/magazine/mag2006/jun2006_report_ashwa_01.htm

Benefits of Ashwagandha: Promoting Sexual Health and Immune Booster | Conscious Life News
http://consciouslifenews.com/benefits-ashwagandha-promoting-sexual-health-immune-booster/#

Ashwagandha | Whole Health Chicago
http://www.wholehealthchicago.com/875/ashwagandha/

Ashwagandha | Organic Herbal Supplements - Mercola.com
http://organicindia.mercola.com/herbal-supplements/ashwagandha.aspx

Ashwagandha Testosterone » Herbal Booster « Withania somnifera
http://anabolicmen.com/ashwagandha-testosterone/

Forty percent more testosterone with Ashwagandha | Ergo Log
http://www.ergo-log.com/withaniasomnifera.html

Ashwagandha extract may suppress cortisol; increased testosterone - Nutrient Journal
http://nutrientjournal.com/ashwagandha-extrac-may-suppress-cortisol-increased-testosterone/

Is The Female Menstrual Cycle Natural? | News | D Herbs
http://dherbs.com/news/4463/4669/Is-The-Female-Menstrual-Cycle-Natural/d,ai.html#.UsI3VNLFqCY

5 Ways that Stress Causes Hypothyroid Symptoms | Chris Kresser
http://chriskresser.com/5-ways-that-stress-causes-hypothyroid-symptoms

The Natural Path to Hormonal Wellness, Part 1 by Katarina Nolte
Pages: 201 (23,609 words); Copyright © 2014 by Katarina Nolte.
All rights reserved. http://katarinanolte.com/ July 2014

Natural proven ways to raise testosterone - Bodybuilding.com Forums
http://forum.bodybuilding.com/showthread.php?t=128535663

Get pregnant? How to get pregnant naturally
http://www.getpregnanttobepregnant.blogspot.com/

Man Up: Boost Your Testosterone Level for Health, Power and Confidence | Washington's Blog
http://www.washingtonsblog.com/2012/04/man-up-boost-your-testosterone-level-for-health-power-and-confidence.html

2 - Herbal Aphrodisiacs | In Harmony Herbs
http://www.inharmonyherbs.com/articles/95-herbal-aphrodisiacs.html

Kama Rani for Female Arousal | Kamarani
http://www.kamarani.com/?aff=dreddyclinic

Herbs For low libido Herbal Remedies | Annie's Remedy
http://www.anniesremedy.com/chart_remedy.php?tag=libido

Top herbs for hormonal balance | Delicious Living
www.m.deliciousliving.com/supplements/top-herbs-hormonal-balance

What herbs help to build muscle - WikiAnswers
http://wiki.answers.com/Q/What_herbs_help_to_build_muscle

The appearance of cellulite is often a sign of a congested lymph system. Massage the areas of your body where the cellulite exists, as well as the lymph nodes in your groin to help improve the condition.
How to Cleanse the Lymph System: 9 Steps (with Pictures) | Wiki How
http://www.wikihow.com/Cleanse-the-Lymph-System

The Natural Path to Hormonal Wellness, Part 1 by Katarina Nolte
Pages: 201 (23,609 words); Copyright © 2014 by Katarina Nolte.
All rights reserved. http://katarinanolte.com/ July 2014

AVENA SATIVA

Oat grass has been used traditionally for medicinal purposes, including to help balance the menstrual cycle, treat dysmenorrhoea, and for osteoporosis and urinary tract infections.
Oat - Wikipedia, the free encyclopedia
http://en.wikipedia.org/wiki/Oat

Avena sativa, also known as green oats or oat straw, has been in use since ancient times as a women's herbal remedy for various hormonal issues and is commonly found in natural erectile dysfunction and muscle building concoctions.

It should be noted that the current cultural gender bias leads to the impression that women and men require opposing properties when it comes to herbs and supplements for optimal health and functioning. Avena sativa is one example of many proving such assumptions to be incorrect.

Avena sativa is an adaptogen assisting the mind-body system in regaining overall homeostasis, including hormonal balance.
Avena sativa combines well with nettle (urtica diotica) and should be cycled — 3 weeks on and 1 week off, or 2 weeks on 2 weeks off — or used irregularly (1-2 times/week).

54

The Natural Path to Hormonal Wellness, Part 1 by Katarina Nolte
Pages: 201 (23,609 words); Copyright © 2014 by Katarina Nolte.
All rights reserved. http://katarinanolte.com/ July 2014

AVENA SATIVA USES

- Sexual and reproductive function
- Stress management (adrenal/thyroid health)
- Neuroprotective and neuroregenerative
- Rest and recovery support, athletic and otherwise
- Longevity, antiaging, regeneration, and rejuvenation
- Gastrointestinal health
- Connective tissue strengthening

Avena sativa contains beta-sitosterol, betaine, quercetin, stigmasterol, B vitamins, vitamins A and E, magnesium, calcium, manganese, zinc, selenium, and iron.

Avena sativa can be purchased whole, crushed, ground, or in capsule form.

Avena sativa can be enjoyed as a tea, tincture, essential oil, extract, or infusion.

Traditional preparation: tea, extract.

NOTE

Do not consume with sugar or sweeteners. Sugar and sweeteners are counter effective to hormonal balance.

The Natural Path to Hormonal Wellness, Part 1 by Katarina Nolte
Pages: 201 (23,609 words); Copyright © 2014 by Katarina Nolte.
All rights reserved. http://katarinanolte.com/ July 2014

LEARN MORE

Gynecological Herbs | Prickly Pear Junction
http://www.pricklypearjunction.com/interactions/Herb_Groups/Gynecological.htm

10 foods that lower testosterone levels | Iron Magazine Forums
http://www.ironmagazineforums.com/diet-nutrition/31148-10-foods-lower-testosterone-levels.html

10 Supps You Never Thought of - Muscle & Fitness
http://www.muscleandfitness.com/news-and-features/galleries/nutrition/10-supps-you-never-thought

Super Male Vitality | Infowars Shop
http://www.infowarsshop.com/Super-Male-Vitality_p_1227.html

Testosterone support - Nutrition Express Articles
http://www.nutritionexpress.com/showarticle.aspx?articleid=753

Avena Sativa - Oats Benefits & Information | Herb Wisdom
http://www.herbwisdom.com/herb-avena-sativa.html

Oatstraw Extract Medicinal Uses Benefits | Annie's Remedy
http://www.anniesremedy.com/herb_detail273.php

Avena Tinctures As Nerve Tonics | Annie's Remedy
http://www.anniesremedy.com/chart_remedy.php?rem_ID=530

Natural Antidepressants Depression Herbs | Annie's Remedy
http://www.anniesremedy.com/chart_remedy_depression.php

Traditional Herbs of the Ancient Middle East | Annie's Remedy
http://www.anniesremedy.com/medicinal_plants_middleeast.php

The Natural Path to Hormonal Wellness, Part 1 by Katarina Nolte
Pages: 201 (23,609 words); Copyright © 2014 by Katarina Nolte.
All rights reserved. http://katarinanolte.com/ July 2014

Stigmasterol is very similar in chemical structure to testosterone, and it's believed that it binds to the same receptors in the body that testosterone binds to, causing an effect similar to that of testosterone.
A Man in Full | Muscle & Body Magazine
http://www.muscleandbodymag.com/a-man-in-full/

The Natural Path to Hormonal Wellness, Part 1 by Katarina Nolte
Pages: 201 (23,609 words); Copyright © 2014 by Katarina Nolte.
All rights reserved. http://katarinanolte.com/ July 2014

CATUABA

*Early human diets were rich in phytosterols,
providing as much as 1 g/d; however, the typical
Western diet today is relatively low in phytosterols.*
**Phytosterols | Linus Pauling Institute at Oregon
State University**
http://lpi.oregonstate.edu/infocenter/phytochemicals/
sterols/

Catuaba is a Central and South American
rainforest plant in the coca family and may
therefore possess stimulant properties but is not a
narcotic. Stimulant effects are often misinterpreted
as being health supportive.
As with tribulus terrestris and other herbs, quality
can be of concern when it comes to its
effectiveness. One should opt for pesticide-free,
organic, wild harvested catuaba.

Catuaba is traditionally used for female and male
pleasure enhancement due to its positive effects on
circulation and dopamine levels.

Catuaba combines well with muira puama and
should be cycled — 3 weeks on and 1 week off, or 2
weeks on 2 weeks off — or used irregularly (1-2
times/week).

The Natural Path to Hormonal Wellness, Part 1 by Katarina Nolte
Pages: 201 (23,609 words); Copyright © 2014 by Katarina Nolte.
All rights reserved. http://katarinanolte.com/ July 2014

CATUABA USES

- Sexual and reproductive function
- Immune system support
- Stress management
- Rest and recovery support, athletic and otherwise
- Longevity, antiaging, regeneration, and rejuvenation
- Neuroprotective and neuroregenerative
- Vitality, energy, spirit, and stamina
- Pain alleviation
- Anti-inflammatory, antioxidant, anti-viral, and antibacterial

Catuaba contains phytosterols, tannins, and flavonoids.

The medicinal catuaba bark is used as a tincture, decoction, capsule, infusion, tea, and extract.

Traditional preparation: tea, tincture.

NOTE

Do not consume with sugar or sweeteners. Sugar and sweeteners are counter effective to hormonal balance.

LEARN MORE

Catuaba Bark Medicinal Uses Benefits | Annie's Remedy
http://www.anniesremedy.com/herb_detail420.php

Catuaba bark is used for a variety of problems – from enhancing the erection to helping with depression and fatigue. | Ageless.co.za
http://www.ageless.co.za/herb-catuaba.htm

Catuaba supplement bark extract aphrodisiac herb, side effects | Ray Sahelian
http://www.raysahelian.com/catuaba.html

Catuaba Bark Testosterone » Natural Male Hormone Booster From Amazon! | Anabolic Men
http://anabolicmen.com/catuaba-bark-testosterone/

The Testosterone Report: Catuaba Bark
http://thetestosteronereport.blogspot.com/2008/05/catuaba-bark.html

Tropical Plant Database File for: Catuaba - Erythroxylum cvatuaba | Rain Tree
http://www.rain-tree.com/catuaba.htm#.U32Tw9JdWSo

Sustainable Rainforest Products | Rain Tree
http://rain-tree.com/product.htm#.U2Bs8YFdVv4

Antidepressant-like effects of Trichilia catigua (Catuaba) extract: evidence for dopaminergic-mediated mechanisms. [Psychopharmacology (Berl). 2005] - PubMed - NCBI
http://www.ncbi.nlm.nih.gov/pubmed/15991001

Different methods can be used on the same plant to get different results. Different parts of the same plant can also yield components intended to treat rather different issues (e.g. Evening Primrose is used internally to lower cholesterol and externally to treat eczema).

TESTOSTERONE NATION | My 'Test Boosting' Tincture - Page 1
http://tnation.t-nation.com/free_online_forum/diet_performance_nutrition_supplements/my_test_boosting_tincture

The Natural Path to Hormonal Wellness, Part 1 by Katarina Nolte
Pages: 201 (23,609 words); Copyright © 2014 by Katarina Nolte.
All rights reserved. http://katarinanolte.com/ July 2014

EPILOBIUM

There are only two prescription testosterone products in the world for women, TestoMeds' AndroFeme and the Intrinsa patch, which was only available in Europe and is now discontinued. AndroFeme is licensed for export from Australia, where TestoMeds products are manufactured, making it the only such cream available for American women.
Treat Low Testosterone and Progesterone Deficiencies with Bioidentical Hormone Replacement Creams – BET SHEMESH, Israel, Aug. 2, 2013 – PRNewswire
http://www.prnewswire.com/news-releases/treat-low-testosterone-and-progesterone-deficiencies-with-bioidentical-hormone-replacement-creams-from-testomeds-218106121.html

Epilobium (fireweed) is a common medicinal herb found all over the world.

Epilobium is said to cause a reduction in 5-alpha-reductase, thereby limiting testosterone to dehydrotestosterone (DHT) conversion. DHT is associated with hairloss, prostate disease, and other health issues.

Epilobium is also believed to inhibit aromatase, thereby reducing the conversion of testosterone to estrogen. The enzyme aromatase is known to rise with age and fat accumulation.

The Natural Path to Hormonal Wellness, Part 1 by Katarina Nolte
Pages: 201 (23,609 words); Copyright © 2014 by Katarina Nolte.
All rights reserved. http://katarinanolte.com/ July 2014

Epilobium should be cycled — 3 weeks on and 1 week off, or 2 weeks on 2 weeks off — or used irregularly (1-2 times/week).

EPILOBIUM USES

- Sexual and reproductive function
- Weight management
- Immune system support
- Anti-cancer, anti-tumor, antifungal, and antiviral

Epilobium contains beta carotene, vitamin C, quercetin and tannins.

Epilobium is consumed raw, in powder form, as a capsule, tea, extract, decoction, or tincture.

Traditional preparation: cold infusion, extract.

NOTE

Do not consume with sugar or sweeteners. Sugar and sweeteners are counter effective to hormonal balance.

LEARN MORE

5-alpha reductase - Wikipedia, the free encyclopedia
http://en.wikipedia.org/wiki/5-alpha_reductase
5-alpha-reductase inhibitor - Wikipedia, the free encyclopedia
http://en.wikipedia.org/wiki/5-alpha-reductase_inhibitor#Herbs_and_other_inhibitors

Inhibition of 5α-Reductase and Aromatase by the Ellagitannins Oenothein A and Oenothein B from Epilobium Species – Thieme E-Journals - Planta Medica
https://www.thieme-connect.com/ejournals/abstract/10.1055/s-2006-957624

Epilobium.com
http://www.epilobium.com/

Natural Products as Aromatase Inhibitors | ncbi.nlm.nih.gov
http://www.ncbi.nlm.nih.gov/pmc/articles/PMC3074486/

Fireweed Medicinal Uses Benefits | Annie's Remedy
http://www.anniesremedy.com/herb_detail98.php

Antitumor activity of oenothein B, a unique macrocyclic ellagitannin. [Jpn J Cancer Res. 1993] - PubMed - NCBI
http://www.ncbi.nlm.nih.gov/pubmed/8449833

Oenothein
http://www.raysahelian.com/oenothein.html

Effect of oenothein B, a cyclic dimeric ellagitannin isolated from Epilobium angustifolium, on the antiviral responses of innate lymphocytes. (P4365) -- Ramstead et al. 190 (1001): 183.18 -- The Journal of Immunology
http://www.jimmunol.org/cgi/content/meeting_abstract/190/1_MeetingAbstracts/183.18

Extracts from Epilobium sp. Herbs, Their Components and Gut Microbiota Metabolites of Epilobium Ellagitannins, Urolithins, Inhibit Hormone-Dependent Prostate Cancer Cells-(LNCaP) Proliferation and PSA Secretion. - ResearchGate
http://www.researchgate.net/publication/235717816_Extracts_from_Epilobium_sp._Herbs_Their_Components_and_Gut_Microbiota_Metabolites_of_Epilobium_Ellagitannins_Urolithins_Inhibit_Hormone-Dependent_Prostate_Cancer_Cells-(LNCaP)_Proliferation_and_PSA_Secretion

Epilobium - Wikipedia, the free encyclopedia

http://en.wikipedia.org/wiki/Epilobium#Use_by_humans

The next time you step out of the shower and reach for your bath towel, stop and stand up straight. Now look down: If you can see your testicles, congratulations, Mr. T. But if a big belly is blocking the view of your jewels, it's likely that your testosterone levels aren't anywhere near what they could be.

Testosterone, Hormones, and Weight Loss | Men's Health

http://www.menshealth.com/weight-loss/improve-your-testosterone

The Natural Path to Hormonal Wellness, Part 1 by Katarina Nolte
Pages: 201 (23,609 words); Copyright © 2014 by Katarina Nolte.
All rights reserved. http://katarinanolte.com/ July 2014

FENUGREEK

Low protein diets have been shown to decrease activity of something called cytochrome P450 that detoxifies estrogen.

10 Ways To Lower Estrogen Toxic Load | Poliquin Article

http://www.poliquingroup.com/ArticlesMultimedia/Articles/Article/801/10_Ways_To_Lower_Estrogen_Toxic_Load_.aspx

Fenugreek is a Middle Eastern herb used medicinally and consumed as a spice and a vegetable.

Fenugreek has traditionally been used to improve fertility.

Fenugreek contains phytoestrogens. Phytoestroens, when consumed in modcrate amounts tend to occupy estrogen receptors. Phytoestrogens are slightly weaker than endogenous estrogens and considerably weaker than industrial xenoestrogens, and therefore present a healthier alternative to the status quo which is that most humans today are loaded with hyper estrogenic xenoestrogens.

For best results, fenugreek should be used in combination with adaptogenic herbs and dietary and supplemental aromatase inhibitors.

Fenugreek should be cycled — 3 weeks on and 1 week off, or 2 weeks on 2 weeks off — or used irregularly (1-2 times/week).

65

The Natural Path to Hormonal Wellness, Part 1 by Katarina Nolte
Pages: 201 (23,609 words); Copyright © 2014 by Katarina Nolte.
All rights reserved. http://katarinanolte.com/ July 2014

FENUGREEK USES

- Sexual and reproductive function
- Blood sugar balance
- Rest and recovery support, athletic and otherwise
- Weight management
- Connective tissue strengthening
- Longevity, antiaging, regeneration, and rejuvenation
- Vitality, energy, and stamina

Fenugreek contains beta-sitosterol, diosgenin, quercetin, rutin, saponin, B vitamins, vitamin C, essential fatty acids, amino acids, magnesium, calcium, selenium, zinc, manganese, and iron.

Fenugreek is consumed as a tea, capsule, powder (ground), and extract.

Traditional preparation: decoction.

NOTE

Do not consume with sugar or sweeteners. Sugar and sweeteners are counter effective to hormonal balance.

LEARN MORE

Fenugreek increases testosterone. And it smells. | Rob Thoburn
http://robthoburn.wordpress.com/2011/02/05/fenugreek-increases-testosterone-and-it-smells/

Estrogen overload - How environment and lifestyle contribute to hormonal imbalance while devastating the health of both men and women | Natural News
http://www.naturalnews.com/040811_hormonal_imbalance_progesterone_surplus_estrogen.html

7 Natural Testosterone Boosters – Vitamins, Minerals and Herbs That Increase Testosterone | Fitness and Power
http://www.fitnessandpower.com/bodybuilding-supplements/7-natural-testosterone-boosters-vitamins-minerals-and-herbs-that-increase-testosterone

Fenugreek boosts bodybuilders' testosterone | Ergo Log
http://www.ergo-log.com/pasio.index.html

Fenugreek - Wikipedia, the free encyclopedia
http://en.wikipedia.org/wiki/Fenugreek

Effects of Torabolic supplementation on strength and body composition during an 8-week resistance training program | ncbi.nlm.nih.gov
http://www.ncbi.nlm.nih.gov/pmc/articles/PMC3313094/

Fenugreek boosts growth hormone emission too | Ergo Log
http://www.ergo-log.com/fenugreekgrowthhormone.html

Fenugreek improves effect of creatine more than carbs | Ergo Log
http://www.ergo-log.com/fenugreekcreatine.html

Testosterone Herbs | Peak Testosterone
http://www.peaktestosterone.com/Testosterone_Herbs.aspx

13 Ways to Boost Your Testosterone - MuscleMag
http://www.musclemag.com/muscle-building/13-ways-to-boost-your-testosterone/#.UtsGrNLTmt8

Chew on this: Everything You Don't Want to Know about Fast Food - Eric Schlosser, Charles Wilson - Google Books
http://books.google.com/books/about/Chew_on_this.html?id=XdkZb4tiIZUC

Fenugreek saponins resemble cholesterol, and human studies show that they can lower levels of cholesterol and triglycerides, compounds associated with heart disease.

Saponin: Natural Steroids | Mother Earth Living

http://www.motherearthliving.com/health-and-wellness/inside-plants-herbs-can-mimic-human-hormones-12-herbs-can-mimic-human-hormones.aspx?PageId=2#ArticleContent

The Natural Path to Hormonal Wellness, Part 1 by Katarina Nolte
Pages: 201 (23,609 words); Copyright © 2014 by Katarina Nolte.
All rights reserved. http://katarinanolte.com/ July 2014

FORSKOLIN

In women, testosterone levels are at their peak from age 21 to 35. At age 40 a woman has only 50% of the Testosterone that she had at age 21.
Natural Progesterone, Diosgenin, Phyto-Progesterone, Phyto-estrogen, HRT │ Ask Dr Helen
http://www.askdrhelen.com/bioidentical/medicalarchive/thyroid.html

Coleus Forskohlii (Forskolin) is a plant belonging to the mint family, traditionally used in Indian Ayurveda for thyroid, heart, and respiratory issues.

Forskolin may stimulate the production of progesterone and should be cycled —1 week on 3 weeks off, or 2 weeks on 2 weeks off — or used irregularly (1-2 times/week).

FORSKOLIN USES

- Neuroprotective and neuroregenerative
- Weight management
- Longevity, antiaging, regeneration, and rejuvenation
- Vitality, energy, and stamina
- Connective tissue strengthening
- Rest and recovery support, athletic and otherwise
- Sexual and reproductive function
- Cardiovascular health
- Respiratory health
- Gastrointestinal health
- Stress management (adrenal/thyroid health)

- Anti-inflammatory, anti-cancer, anti-tumor, antioxidant, anti-allergy, antibacterial, antiviral

Forskolin contains stigmasterol.

Forskolin can be consumed as a tea, capsule, powder (ground), and extract.

Traditional preparation: extract.

NOTE

Do not consume with sugar or sweeteners. Sugar and sweeteners are counter effective to hormonal balance.

LEARN MORE

Forskolin - Wikipedia, the free encyclopedia
http://en.wikipedia.org/wiki/Forskolin
Forskolin Supplements & Products at Bodybuilding.com - Lowest Prices on Forskolin!
http://www.bodybuilding.com/store/fors.html
Body composition and hormonal adaptations associated with forskolin consumption in overweight and obese men. - PubMed - NCBI
http://www.ncbi.nlm.nih.gov/pubmed/16129715
Forskolin supplement extract | Ray Sahelian
http://www.raysahelian.com/forskolin.html
Ayurveda - Wikipedia, the free encyclopedia
http://en.wikipedia.org/wiki/Ayurveda

Forskolin: Friend or Foe? Stories and Studies About Fat Loss, Lean Gains, Topical Cellulite Treatment, Testosterone, Cancer, Hepatotoxicity, Drug Interactions & More - SuppVersity
http://suppversity.blogspot.com/2012/12/forskolin-friend-or-foe-stories-and.html

T NATION | Burn Fat, Build Muscle With Forskolin
http://www.t-nation.com/supplements/burn-fat-pile-on-muscle-with-forskolin

T NATION | Don't Kill the Messenger
http://www.t-nation.com/free_online_article/sports_body_training_performance_science/dont_kill_the_messenger

Nicotine as anti-aromatase - Bodybuilding.com Forums
http://forum.bodybuilding.com/showthread.php?t=4700003

Adaptogens in Medical Herbalism: Elite Herbs and Natural Compounds for Mastering Stress, Aging, and Chronic Disease - Donald R. Yance, CN, MH, RH(AHG) - Google Books
http://goo.gl/t4m4HY

Luteolin, the anti-oestrogen in celery | Ergo Log
http://www.ergo-log.com/luteolin-anti-oestrogen-in-celery.html

Progesterone, Phytoprogesterones, Phytoprogestogenics | Your Menopause Type
http://www.yourmenopausetype.com/e-news/volume12.html

Androgens (male hormones) are crucial to female fertility, suggests new CHR publication | CHR
http://www.centerforhumanreprod.com/news_androgens_egg_development.html

71

The Natural Path to Hormonal Wellness, Part 1 by Katarina Nolte
Pages: 201 (23,609 words); Copyright © 2014 by Katarina Nolte.
All rights reserved. http://katarinanolte.com/ July 2014

Most women hit their fertile peak between the ages of 23 and 31, though the rate at which women conceive begins to dip slightly in their late 20s. Around age 31, fertility starts to drop more quickly — by about 3 percent per year — until you hit 35 or so. From there, the decline accelerates. "The average 39-year-old woman has half the fertility she had at 31, and between 39 and 42, the chances of conceiving drop by half again," says Adamson.
Fertility 101 | Web MD
http://www.webmd.com/baby/features/fertility-101

The Natural Path to Hormonal Wellness, Part 1 by Katarina Nolte
Pages: 201 (23,609 words); Copyright © 2014 by Katarina Nolte.
All rights reserved. http://katarinanolte.com/ July 2014

FO-TI

Androgen replacement for women is a neglected area of medicine. None of the standard textbooks of medicine, endocrinology, clinical pathology, or pharmacology, which we reviewed, made any mention of androgen deficiency in women.
Testosterone for Women Newsletter | Women's International
http://www.womensinternational.com/connections/testosterone.html

Fo-ti (polygonum multiflorum) is an adaptogenic herb which has been used in China for its many medicinal properties since ancient times.

Fo-ti should be cycled — 3 weeks on and 1 week off, or 2 weeks on 2 weeks off — or used irregularly (1-2 times/week).

FO-TI USES

- Vitality, energy, spirit, and stamina
- Longevity, antiaging, regeneration, and rejuvenation
- Pain alleviation
- Sexual and reproductive function
- Rest and recovery support, athletic and otherwise
- Neuroprotective and neuroregenerative
- Stress management (adrenal/thyroid health)
- Detoxification (liver, kidney, lymph tissues)
- Gastrointestinal health
- Connective tissue strengthening

- Immune system support
- Blood sugar balance
- Anti-inflammatory, antibacterial, antifungal, anti-tumor, anti-cancer, and antioxidant

Fo-ti contains chrysophanol, alkaloids, and zinc.

Fo-ti is consumed in powder form, as a capsule, tea, extract, decoction, or tincture.

Traditional preparation: tea, tincture.

NOTE

Do not consume with sugar or sweeteners. Sugar and sweeteners are counter effective to hormonal balance.

LEARN MORE

Anti-Inflammatory activity of chrysophanol through the suppression of NF-kappaB/caspase-1 activation in vitro and in vivo. [Molecules. 2010] - PubMed - NCBI
http://www.ncbi.nlm.nih.gov/pubmed/20877234
Chrysophanol induces necrosis through the production of ROS and alteration of ATP levels in J5 human liver cancer cells. | ncbi.nlm.nih.gov
http://www.ncbi.nlm.nih.gov/pubmed/20169580
Fo-ti Root Benefits & Information (Polygonum Multiflorum) | Herb Wisdom
http://www.herbwisdom.com/herb-fo-ti-root.html
Fo-Ti Root – Mountain Rose Herbs
https://www.mountainroseherbs.com/products/fo-ti-root/profile

The Natural Path to Hormonal Wellness, Part 1 by Katarina Nolte
Pages: 201 (23,609 words); Copyright © 2014 by Katarina Nolte.
All rights reserved. http://katarinanolte.com/ July 2014

Fo-Ti root is the most effective of the fertility herbs for gray hair reversal. | Secrets of Longevity in Humans
http://www.secrets-of-longevity-in-humans.com/fo-ti-root.html
All about the Adaptogenic Herb Fo-Ti and It's Many Health Benefits | Underground Health Reporter
http://undergroundhealthreporter.com/adaptogenic-herb-foti-for-longevity-and-energy/#axzz34JdKyavM
Fo-Ti Root He-shou-wu Medicinal Uses Benefits | Annie's Remedy
http://www.anniesremedy.com/herb_detail313.php
Brazilian Journal of Medical and Biological Research - An extract of Polygonum multiflorum protects against free radical damage induced by ultraviolet B irradiation of the skin
http://www.scielo.br/scielo.php?pid=s0100-879x2006000900005&script=sci_arttext&tlng=en

One of the earliest reports showing an association between decreased sexual desire and decreased testosterone in women was published in 1959, but acceptance of this association has been slow. However, more evidence now shows that many women – pre-menopausal and post-menopausal – do suffer from androgen deficiency. Because the symptoms of such a deficiency resemble those of depression, misdiagnosis and lack of treatment are common.
Testosterone insufficiency in women: fact or fiction? » Sexual Medicine » BUMC
http://www.bumc.bu.edu/sexualmedicine/publications/testosterone-insufficiency-in-women-fact-or-fiction/

The Natural Path to Hormonal Wellness, Part 1 by Katarina Nolte
Pages: 201 (23,609 words); Copyright © 2014 by Katarina Nolte.
All rights reserved. http://katarinanolte.com/ July 2014

GINSENG

Very few women over 44 are still fertile.
Age and Female Infertility, Fertility Tests of Egg Supply | Advanced Fertility
http://www.advancedfertility.com/age.htm

Ginseng is an ancient adaptogenic herb native to China and North America and is one of the main aphrodisiac herbs used in Traditional Chinese Medicine.

The herb eleuthero, sometimes called 'Siberian Ginseng', has similar properties as (Panax) ginseng.

Ginseng should be cycled — 3 weeks on and 1 week off, or 2 weeks on 2 weeks off — or used irregularly (1-2 times/week).

GINSENG USES

- Vitality, energy, spirit, and stamina
- Sexual and reproductive function
- Rest and recovery support, athletic and otherwise
- Stress management (adrenal/thyroid health)
- Pain alleviation
- Immune system support
- Longevity, antiaging, regeneration, and rejuvenation
- Cardiovascular health
- Blood sugar balance
- Detoxification (liver, kidney, lymph tissues)

- Neuroprotective and neuroregenerative

Ginseng contains beta-sitosterol, saponin, stigmasterol, vitamin C, B vitamins, magnesium, calcium, zinc, manganese, and iron.

The medicinal ginseng root and leaves can be consumed as a tea, capsule, powder, extract, essential oil, tincture, and infusion.

Traditional preparation: tea, decoction.

NOTE

Do not consume with sugar or sweeteners. Sugar and sweeteners are counter effective to hormonal balance.

LEARN MORE

Dr. Wright's Most Powerful Anti-Aging Breakthroughs Jonathan V. Wright, M.D.
https://images.web-purchases.com/Library-1500034/600RNAHPDF_NAHUpsellPremiums.pdf
Eleutherococcus senticosus - Wikipedia, the free encyclopedia
http://en.wikipedia.org/wiki/Eleutherococcus_senticosus
Top 5 Proven Herbs to Increase Testosterone Naturally | Atl Night Spots
http://www.atlnightspots.com/top-5-proven-herbs-to-increase-testosterone-naturally/

A 2002 study of 782 couples did find decreased fertility for older men; in specific, 35-39 year old women whose male partners were the same age had a probability of pregnancy under certain conditions of 0.29, but if the male partner was five years older the probability decreased to 0.18.

Paternal age effect - Wikipedia, the free encyclopedia

http://en.wikipedia.org/wiki/Paternal_age_effect

The Natural Path to Hormonal Wellness, Part 1 by Katarina Nolte
Pages: 201 (23,609 words); Copyright © 2014 by Katarina Nolte.
All rights reserved. http://katarinanolte.com/ July 2014

HORNY GOAT WEED

Being a female and being in balance is possible and our natural state.
HANS - Natural Hormone Balance
http://www.hans.org/magazine/812/Natural-Hormone-Balance.html

Horny goat weed (epimedium) is an ancient Chinese aphrodisiac herb which shares some chemical similarities with the erectile dysfunction pharmaceutical sildenafil (Viagra).

Horny goat weed is traditionally used for libido and female problems.

Horny goat weed should be cycled — 3 weeks on and 1 week off, or 2 weeks on 2 weeks off — or used irregularly (1-2 times/week).

HORNY GOAT WEED USES

- Connective tissue strengthening
- Longevity, antiaging, regeneration, and rejuvenation
- Vitality, energy, spirit, and stamina
- Sexual and reproductive function
- Neuroprotective and neuroregenerative
- Stress management (adrenal health)
- Rest and recovery support, athletic and otherwise
- Weight management
- Gastrointestinal health
- Cardiovascular health

- Respiratory health
- Chronic disease prevention and treatment
- Anti-inflammatory, antioxidant, anti-cancer, and anti-tumor

Horny goat weed is rich in flavonoids which makes it a potent antioxidant supplement. Antioxidants are known to improve testosterone levels.

Horny goat weed (leaf) can be consumed as a tea, whole, capsule, powder, extract, tincture, and infusion.

Traditional preparation: tea.

NOTE

Do not consume with sugar or sweeteners. Sugar and sweeteners are counter effective to hormonal balance.

LEARN MORE

Making Goat Weed Tinctures and Teas | Horny Goat Weed Farm
http://hornygoatweedfarm.com/makinggoatweedteasandtinctures.html
Icariin | Peak Testosterone
http://www.peaktestosterone.com/Icariin.aspx
4 Things to Do and 3 Things to Stop to Naturally Increase Your Testosterone | Breaking Muscle
http://breakingmuscle.com/mens-fitness/4-things-to-do-and-3-things-to-stop-to-naturally-increase-your-testosterone

50 Foods That Boost Testosterone Naturally » High Testosterone Diet | Anabolic Men
http://anabolicmen.com/50-foods-that-boost-testosterone-levels/

Flavonoid in Horny Goat Weed boosts testosterone | Ergo Log
http://www.ergo-log.com/icariintestosterone.html

Female Libido | Naturally Increase Female Libido | Natural Wellbeing
http://www.naturalwellbeing.com/products/female-libido-1

Testosterone Estrogen | Peak Testosterone
http://www.peaktestosterone.com/Estrogen.aspx

6 Herbs That'll Make Your Orgasms Mind-Blowing | Your Tango
http://www.yourtango.com/experts/rn-mh-dawn-gates/natural-ways-have-more-fulfilling-orgasm

Vegan men tended to have significantly higher testosterone levels than both vegetarians and meateaters.

Vegan Men: More Testosterone But Less Cancer | Nutrition Facts
http://nutritionfacts.org/2013/02/12/less-cancer-in-vegan-men-despite-more-testosterone/

The Natural Path to Hormonal Wellness, Part 1 by Katarina Nolte
Pages: 201 (23,609 words); Copyright © 2014 by Katarina Nolte.
All rights reserved. http://katarinanolte.com/ July 2014

LONGJACK

99.9% of hormones in the body are regulated by a process called negative feedback. What this means is that the presence of a hormone actually turns off the production of that hormone. Homeostasis – the ideal state of the body – uses negative feedback to monitor most bodily functions. When levels drop, the body increases production of the hormone who's levels have just dropped. All sex hormones use negative feedback to maintain healthy levels. Each person will have a different "set point" that the body uses as a reference for homeostasis. Drop below the set point, and you will produce more (lets say) testosterone until you reach that "set point."

Tongkat Ali and Raising the Testosterone Thermostat - Pine Pollen | RAW Forest Foods

http://www.rawforestfoodsblog.com/tongkat-ali-and-raising-the-testosterone-thermostat/

Longjack (tongkat ali) is an ancient adaptogenic tropical herb native to Southeast Asia.

Longjack is traditionally used against malaria and as a libido enhancer and is consumed as a food and a spice.

Quality can be of concern. One should opt for pesticide-free, organic, wild harvested eurycoma longfolia jack.

Longjack should be cycled — 3 weeks on and 1 week off, or 2 weeks on 2 weeks off — or used irregularly (1-2 times/week).

LONGJACK USES

- Sexual and reproductive function
- Stress management (adrenal health)
- Longevity, antiaging, regeneration, and rejuvenation
- Vitality, energy, spirit, and stamina
- Rest and recovery support, athletic and otherwise
- Connective tissue strengthening
- Neuroprotective and neuroregenerative
- Immune system support
- Respiratory health
- Blood sugar balance
- Antibacterial, antiviral, anti-fever, and anti-cancer

Longjack contains saponins, lignans, and alkaloids.

The medicinal longjack root can be consumed as a tea, capsule, tincture, infusion, or extract.

Traditional preparation: decoction.

NOTE

Do not consume with sugar or sweeteners. Sugar and sweeteners are counter effective to hormonal balance.

LEARN MORE

Eurycoma longifolia - Wikipedia, the free encyclopedia
http://en.wikipedia.org/wiki/Eurycoma_longifolia
Effect of Tongkat Ali on stress hormones and psychological mood state in moderately stressed subjects | ncbi.nlm.nih.gov
http://www.ncbi.nlm.nih.gov/pmc/articles/PMC3669033/
Eurycoma Longifolia Benefits | Zhion
http://www.zhion.com/herb/Eurycoma_Longifolia_Benefits.html
Ageing Male Symptoms (AMS) Questionnaire | HormoneSolutions.com.au
http://www.hormonesolutions.com.au/content/testosterone-cream-for-men/AMS-self-assessment.php
The Aging Males' Symptoms (AMS) scale: Update and compilation of international versions | ncbi.nlm.nih.gov
http://www.ncbi.nlm.nih.gov/pmc/articles/PMC155679/
Eurycoma longifolia - Wikipedia, the free encyclopedia
http://en.wikipedia.org/wiki/Eurycoma_longifolia
How Eurycoma longifolia boosts testosterone levels | Ergo Log
http://www.ergo-log.com/how-eurycoma-longifolia-boosts-testosterone-levels.html
Weltiner - 6 capsules: Souvenirs de Nouvelle-Zélande | Shop New Zealand
http://www.shopnewzealand.co.nz/fr/cp/Weltiner
Raising Testosterone Levels With Zinc Supplements and a High Zinc Diet | Muscle Health Fitness
http://www.muscle-health-fitness.com/raising-testosterone-levels.html/

Muscle building effect of Tongkat Ali shown in animal study | Ergo Log
http://www.ergo-log.com/tongkatanabolic.html
Aphrodisiac Tongkat Ali boosts testosterone level | Ergo Log
http://www.ergo-log.com/tongkatalitest.html
How Eurycoma longifolia boosts testosterone levels | Ergo Log
http://www.ergo-log.com/how-eurycoma-longifolia-boosts-testosterone-levels.html
Paleo and Testosterone | Robb Wolf
http://robbwolf.com/2011/11/02/paleo-and-testosterone/
Less cortisol and more testosterone with a daily 200 mg Tongkat Ali | Ergo Log
http://www.ergo-log.com/less-cortisol-more-testosterone-with-a-daily-200-mg-tongkat-ali.html
Tongkat Ali has no effect on prostate | Ergo Log
http://www.ergo-log.com/tongkat-ali-has-no-effect-on-prostate.html
The effect of Tongkat Ali on healthy men | Ergo Log
http://www.ergo-log.com/the-effect-of-tongkat-ali-on-healthy-men.html
Tongkat Ali raises testosterone levels in over-fifties | Ergo Log
http://www.ergo-log.com/tongkat-ali-raises-testosterone-levels-in-over-fifties.html

Viagra erections, just like alprostadil injections or penis pumps, cause blood flow into the male organ, even if the mind has no sexual desire at all.
Tongkat ali testosterone diet - no obesity, no migraine - but libido - sexual desires make life worth living
http://www.tongkatali.org/

The Natural Path to Hormonal Wellness, Part 1 by Katarina Nolte
Pages: 201 (23,609 words); Copyright © 2014 by Katarina Nolte.
All rights reserved. http://katarinanolte.com/ July 2014

MACA

Maca naturally contains DIM (Diindolylmethane), an indole phytochemical that can be isolated from compounds found in cruciferous vegetables such as broccoli, Brussels sprouts and cabbage. DIM has been found in animal and human studies to greatly improve hormone balance in both men and women, as well as to protect against some forms of cancer.
The Benefits Of Maca Root Supplementation for Athletes and Bodybuilders | Muscle Health Fitness
http://www.muscle-health-fitness.com/benefits-of-maca-root.html/

Maca is a South American root plant in the cruciferous vegetable family, traditionally used for female problems, and as a fertility and immunity booster.

Maca is a feel-good staple food in Peru.

As with tribulus terrestris and other herbs, quality can be of concern when it comes to its effectiveness. One should opt for pesticide-free, organic, wild harvested maca.

Maca is an adaptogen and as such it helps the mind-body system regain homeostasis. If successful, it may lead to hormonal balance and proportionately higher levels of bioavailable (free) testosterone, among other mild improvements in overall wellbeing.

Maca, being a vegetable, doesn't necessarily have to be cycled.

MACA USES

- Vitality, energy, spirit, and stamina
- Rest and recovery support, athletic and otherwise
- Sexual and reproductive function
- Stress management (thyroid/adrenal health)
- Immune system support
- Longevity, antiaging, regeneration, and rejuvenation
- Gastrointestinal health
- Blood sugar balance
- Neuroprotective and neuroregenerative
- Anti-inflammatory and antioxidant

Maca contains amino acids, phytosterols, manganese, zinc, iodine, and iron.

Maca root can be consumed in powder form, as a tea, capsule, spice, tincture, infusion, or extract.

Traditional preparation: cooked food ingredient.
NOTE

Do not consume with sugar or sweeteners. Sugar and sweeteners are counter effective to hormonal balance.

LEARN MORE

Superfoods – Maca: The Queen of the Cruciferous Vegetables | Healthy Creatures
http://healthycreatures.com/superfoods-maca/
Vitamins and Minerals in Maca Root Powder - Indigo International
http://indigointernational.org/vitamins-and-minerals-in-maca-root-powder/
Maca Root: A Compelling True Adaptogen Affects the Body and Mind | Natural News
http://www.naturalnews.com/029101_maca_root_adaptogens.html#
Fighting Exercise Induced Inflammation by Dr. William Wong | Totality of Being
http://www.totalityofbeing.com/FramelessPages/Articles/exercise_inflammation.html
First case report of testosterone assay-interference in a female taking maca (Lepidium meyenii) -- Srikugan et al. 2011 -- BMJ Case Reports
http://casereports.bmj.com/content/2011/bcr.01.2011.3781.abstract
Patent WO2001015713A1 - Maca and antler for augmenting testosterone levels - Google Patents
http://goo.gl/k3R49k
The Hormone Effect - Every Woman's Health Issue | HealthPost.co.nz
http://www.healthpost.co.nz/the-hormone-effect-every-womans-health-issue
Testosterone: Natural Methods to Improve Vitality, Sexual Function, and Prostate Health - Life Extension
http://www.lef.org/magazine/mag2008/dec2008_Natural-Methods-to-Improve-Testosterone-Sexual-Function-Prostate-Health_01.htm
Picea abies - Wikipedia, the free encyclopedia
http://en.wikipedia.org/wiki/Picea_abies#Other_uses

The Real Reason Men Lose Their Hair | Totality of Being
http://www.totalityofbeing.com/FramelessPages/Articles/real_reason_men_lose_hair.htm

Tropical Plant Database entry for: Maca- Lepidium meyenii
http://www.rain-tree.com/maca.htm#.U7O3BpRdWSo

Hudson's Guide: Bioidentical Testosterone | FTM Guide
http://www.ftmguide.org/bioidenticalt.html

Paleo for Women | Phytoestrogens in the Body: How Soy Interferes with Natural Hormone Balance
http://www.paleoforwomen.com/phytoestrogens-estrogens-and-estrogen-receptors/

Paleo for Women | Low on Progesterone? Why Stress Reduction Might Be the Only Way to Hack It
http://www.paleoforwomen.com/low-on-progesterone-stress-reduction-might-be-the-only-one-way-to-hack-it/

NATURAL PROGESTERONE FOR PCOS | PCOS Diva
http://www.pcosdiva.com/2011/02/natural-progesterone-for-pcos/

Maca Smoothie For Energy & Libido - Incredible Smoothies
http://www.incrediblesmoothies.com/super-smoothies/maca-smoothie-for-energy/

Maca madness green smoothie | Dishing Up the Dirt
http://dishingupthedirt.com/recipes/breakfast/maca-madness-smoothie/

Maca | NavitasNaturals.com
http://navitasnaturals.com/recipes/category/9278/Maca.html

Vegan Recipes with Maca Powder | Feastie
http://www.feastie.com/recipes-diet/vegan/ingredients/maca-powder-11772

Radish - Wikipedia, the free encyclopedia
http://en.wikipedia.org/wiki/Radish

Brassicaceae - Wikipedia, the free encyclopedia
http://en.wikipedia.org/wiki/Brassicaceae

Cruciferous vegetables - Wikipedia, the free encyclopedia
http://en.wikipedia.org/wiki/Cruciferous_vegetables

All About DIM – Diindolylmethane | Energetic Nutrition
http://www.energeticnutrition.com/books/all-about-dim.html

List of root vegetables - Wikipedia, the free encyclopedia
http://en.wikipedia.org/wiki/List_of_root_vegetables

Tuber - Wikipedia, the free encyclopedia
http://en.wikipedia.org/wiki/Tuber

Hormonal Balance for Antiaging | Longevity and Antiaging Secrets
http://www.longevity-and-antiaging-secrets.com/hormonal-balance.html

Increasing Fertility and Maintaining Pregnancy Naturally | Totality of Being
http://www.totalityofbeing.com/FramelessPages/Articles/IncFertility.htm

Inca warriors on the verge of taking a city were forbidden by their generals to take maca so as to protect the women in the city.
Maca makes cyclists faster and hornier | Ergo Log
http://www.ergo-log.com/macafaster.html

90

MUCUNA PRURIENS

Testosterone is vital to bone health/bone mineral density, sexual performance, muscle mass, strength, CHD health, cognition and memory, body mass index and body fat, blood glucose metabolism, energy levels, and feelings of well being and depression. Anemia alleviated, hemoglobin raised.
Natural Hormone Replacement Therapy | A Health
http://www.ahealth.com/content/education_research/published_excerpts/media/HRT.pdf

Mucuna pruriens, also known as velvet bean and kapi kacchu, is a tropical plant native to Africa and Asia. Mucuna pruriens has traditionally been used in India, Brazil and the Caribbean as a libido and fertility booster.

Mucuna pruriens appears to possess adaptogenic and aphrodisiac properties, and is said to raise dopamine levels, luteinizing hormone levels, testosterone and growth hormone levels, while proportionately reducing prolactin and estrogen levels.

Because of its effects on testosterone and growth hormones, mucuna pruriens may support the growth of muscle tissues. And increased dopamine generally leads to an improvement in mood and overall outlook.

Mucuna pruriens may also lead to a rise in adrenaline which suggests stimulant properties.

The Natural Path to Hormonal Wellness, Part 1 by Katarina Nolte
Pages: 201 (23,609 words); Copyright © 2014 by Katarina Nolte.
All rights reserved. http://katarinanolte.com/ July 2014

Mucuna pruriens probably doesn't have to by cycled, but should probably not be consumed daily due to its potentially negative effects on digestion.

MUCUNA PRURIENS USES

- Detoxification (liver, kidney, lymph tissues)
- Neuroprotective and neuroregenerative
- Longevity, antiaging, regeneration, and rejuvenation
- Vitality, energy, spirit, and stamina
- Sexual and reproductive function
- Rest and recovery support, athletic and otherwise
- Stress management

Mucuna pruriens contains amino acids, levodopa (l-dopa), tannins, magnesium, calcium, manganese, zinc, copper, and iron.

Mucuna pruriens bean also contains protease inhibitors like many other beans, grains, nuts, and seeds, which makes it a less than ideal food for those with gastrointestinal issues.

Mucuna pruriens can be consumed in powder form, as a tea, capsule, tincture, infusion, or extract.

Traditional preparation: seed decoction; cooked food.

NOTE

Do not consume with sugar or sweeteners. Sugar and sweeteners are counter effective to hormonal balance.

LEARN MORE

Mucuna pruriens: more testosterone, more LH, less prolactin | Ergo Log
http://www.ergo-log.com/mucunatest.html
Mucuna pruriens - Wikipedia, the free encyclopedia
http://en.wikipedia.org/wiki/Mucuna_pruriens
Cowhage (Mucuna pruriens) | Plant Profiler | Sigma-Aldrich
http://www.sigmaaldrich.com/life-science/nutrition-research/learning-center/plant-profiler/mucuna-pruriens.html
L-DOPA - Wikipedia, the free encyclopedia
http://en.wikipedia.org/wiki/L-DOPA
The Hidden Dangers in Your Whole Grains, Beans, Nuts and Seeds? | Health Beyond Hype
http://www.healthbeyondhype.com/the-hidden-dangers-in-your-whole-grains-beans-nuts-and-seeds-ezp-138.html
Antinutrient - Wikipedia, the free encyclopedia
http://en.wikipedia.org/wiki/Antinutrient
Plants Bite Back | Weston A Price
http://www.westonaprice.org/health-topics/plants-bite-back/
Why You Should Soak Your Grains, Beans, Nuts and Seeds | Wake Up World
http://wakeup-world.com/2012/10/18/why-you-should-soak-your-grains-beans-nuts-and-seeds/

The Natural Path to Hormonal Wellness, Part 1 by Katarina Nolte
Pages: 201 (23,609 words); Copyright © 2014 by Katarina Nolte.
All rights reserved. http://katarinanolte.com/ July 2014

Worldwide testosterone levels are falling at an astronomical rate. It's pure delusion to think living in a completely unnatural environment and ingesting estrogen enhancing chemicals daily will let you keep high levels.

Why Your Testosterone Levels are Lower Than You Think (and what to do about it) │ Bold and Determined

http://boldanddetermined.com/2012/08/19/low-testosterone-levels/

MUIRA PUAMA

The detoxification pathways in modern humans have become burdened to the point of malfunction leading to collapse.

The Real Causes of Estrogen Toxicity - Pine Pollen | RAW Forest Foods

http://www.rawforestfoodsblog.com/understanding-estrogen-detoxification/

Muira puama is a rainforest plant traditionally used in Brazil for its stimulant, aphrodisiac and adaptogenic properties.

Muira puama is traditionally consumed on a regular basis, but would probably be most effective when cycled.

MUIRA PUAMA USES

- Longevity, antiaging, regeneration, and rejuvenation
- Stress management
- Vitality, energy, spirit, and stamina
- Sexual and reproductive function
- Neuroprotective and neuroregenerative
- Cardiovascular health
- Detoxification
- Gastrointestinal health
- Weight management
- Pain alleviation
- Antioxidant and anti-inflammatory

Pages: 201 (23,609 words); Copyright © 2014 by Katarina Nolte.
All rights reserved. http://katarinanolte.com/ July 2014

Muira puama contains alkaloids and beta sitosterol.

Muira puama can be consumed in powder form, as a tea, capsule, tincture, infusion, or extract.

Traditional preparation: hot infusion, tincture.

NOTE

Do not consume with sugar or sweeteners. Sugar and sweeteners are counter effective to hormonal balance.

LEARN MORE

Tropical Plant Database entry for: Muira puama - Ptychopetalum olacoides | Rain Tree
http://www.rain-tree.com/muirapuama.htm#.U5D69XJdWSo
Adaptogenic herbs almost always fall into the category of herbal aphrodisiacs | Secrets of Longevity in Humans
http://www.secrets-of-longevity-in-humans.com/adaptogenic-herbs.html
Ptychopetalum - Wikipedia, the free encyclopedia
http://en.wikipedia.org/wiki/Ptychopetalum
Muira puama (Ptychopetalum olacoides) | Plant Profiler | Sigma-Aldrich
http://www.sigmaaldrich.com/life-science/nutrition-research/learning-center/plant-profiler/ptychopetalum-olacoides.html

The Natural Path to Hormonal Wellness, Part 1 by Katarina Nolte
Pages: 201 (23,609 words); Copyright © 2014 by Katarina Nolte.
All rights reserved. http://katarinanolte.com/ July 2014

Once I went raw paleo I got a surge of testosterone and had a major increase in drive. I have conceived my 4th child after a birthday weekend feast of oysters and pig testicles. (She is due in a few weeks.)

Sex drive on a raw diet? | Raw Paleo Diet Forum
http://www.rawpaleodietforum.com/hot-topics/sex-drive-on-a-raw-diet/

The Natural Path to Hormonal Wellness, Part 1 by Katarina Nolte
Pages: 201 (23,609 words); Copyright © 2014 by Katarina Nolte.
All rights reserved. http://katarinanolte.com/ July 2014

NETTLE

Regular exercise of the major muscles like the thighs, gluteals, or lower legs can help, too.
Care of the Masculine | Naturo Doc
http://www.naturodoc.com/library/hormones/masculine.htm

Nettle is a common herb which grows all over the world and has been used medicinally and as a food ingredient for ages. Nettle possesses some adaptogenic properties.

Nettle seems to be quite a powerful herb and should therefore be cycled.

NETTLE USES

- Stress management (adrenal/thyroid health)
- Immune system support
- Longevity, antiaging, regeneration, and rejuvenation
- Vitality, energy, spirit, and stamina
- Neuroprotective and neuroregenerative
- Connective tissue strengthening
- Detoxification (liver, kidney, lymph tissues)
- Gastrointestinal health
- Cardiovascular health
- Sexual and reproductive function
- Rest and recovery support, athletic and otherwise
- Weight management
- Respiratory health

- Anti-inflammatory, anti-allergy, anti-cancer, anti-viral, anti-bacterial, anti-ulcer, anti-parasitic, and antioxidant

Nettle contains amino acids, vitamin A, B vitamins, vitamin C, vitamin D, vitamin E, vitamin K, acetylcholine, magnesium, calcium, manganese, selenium, chromium, zinc, and iron.

Nettle can be consumed as a food, as well as in powder form, as a tea, capsule, tincture, infusion, or extract.

Traditional preparation: decoction.

NOTE

Do not consume with sugar or sweeteners. Sugar and sweeteners are counter effective to hormonal balance.

LEARN MORE

Urtica dioica - Wikipedia, the free encyclopedia
http://en.wikipedia.org/wiki/Urtica_dioica
Adaptogens And The Many Ways We Dance With Life | Hawthorne Hill Herbs
http://www.hawthornehillherbs.com/node/168
The Stinging Nettle – A paradoxical Green Goddess | The Odinic Rite – Guardians
http://www.odinic-rite.org/Guardians/the-stinging-nettle-a-paradoxical-green-goddess/

Stinging nettle health benefits for home remedies that treat just about everything │ Natural News
http://www.naturalnews.com/036080_stinging_nettles_remedies_arthritis.html

Nettle Leaf and Root Tea Benefits │ Superfoods Scientific Research
http://www.superfoods-scientific-research.com/green-foods/nettle-study-results.html

A chitin-binding lectin from stinging nettle rhizomes with antifungal properties. [Science. 1989] - PubMed - NCBI
http://www.ncbi.nlm.nih.gov/pubmed/17838811

Antioxidant, antimicrobial, antiulcer and analgesic activities of nettle (Urtica dioica L.) │ Science Direct
http://www.sciencedirect.com/science/article/pii/S0378874103003490

How to Increase Testosterone Naturally | The Art of Manliness
http://www.artofmanliness.com/2013/01/18/how-to-increase-testosterone-naturally/

7 Popular Natural Testosterone Enhancers Independently Reviewed │ Muscle Health Fitness
http://www.muscle-health-fitness.com/natural-testosterone-enhancers.html/

Free Testosterone – SHBG │ Peak Testosterone
http://www.peaktestosterone.com/Free_Testosterone_SHBG.aspx

Nettle Root and Androgenic Herbs – YouTube
http://youtu.be/btctGxtyPGw

BIO-IDENTICAL HORMONE REPLACEMENT PROGRAM (BHRT) │ Eternity Medicine
http://www.eternitymedicine.com/Attachments/BHRT%20Male%20Manual%20BMM01_2012.pdf

Enlargement Of Prostate - Enzymes - Juicing - Toxins Of Mercury - Prostate Health │ Nutrition 2000
http://www.nutrition2000.com/prostate_and_health/BPH.asp

Men's Health - Murray Avenue Apothecary
http://www.murrayavenuerx.com/mens-health.html
How low magnesium is affecting your hormonal balance | She Knows
http://www.sheknows.com/health-and-wellness/articles/1009485/more-magnesium-for-hormonal-balance
Aromatase | Naturalpedia
http://www.naturalpedia.com/Aromatase-4.html
High SHBG | Peak Testosterone
http://www.peaktestosterone.com/High_SHBG.aspx
Fertility After Forty - conception - Susun Weed - herbal medicine - women's health - orgasm
http://www.susunweed.com/Article_Fertility_After_Forty.htm
Increase Testosterone | Peak Testosterone
http://www.peaktestosterone.com/How-To-Increase-Testosterone-Naturally.aspx

Nettle leaf is among the most valuable herbal remedies. Because of its many nutrients, stinging nettle is traditionally used as a spring tonic. It is a slow-acting nutritive herb that gently cleanses the body of metabolic wastes.
Medicinal Qualities of Stinging Nettle | Herbal Legacy
http://www.herballegacy.com/Vance_Medicinal.html

The Natural Path to Hormonal Wellness, Part 1 by Katarina Nolte
Pages: 201 (23,609 words); Copyright © 2014 by Katarina Nolte.
All rights reserved. http://katarinanolte.com/ July 2014

PINE POLLEN

> *Pine Pollen contains phenylalanine, which is associated with neurotransmitters in the brain. Phenylalanine stimulates dopamine levels in the brain and is a L-dopa precursor. L-dopa has been known to specifically treat a woman's inability to have an orgasm. Pine Pollen contains arginine, which improves fertility in women and men, as well as, increases growth hormone release.*
> **SurThrival News - How Will Pine Pollen Benefit You?**
> http://www.surthrival.com/news/pine-pollen-benefits/

Pinus missoniana pine tree is native to Eastern Asia where different parts of the plant have traditionally been used for their anti-aging and adaptogenic properties. Its pollen contains comparatively high levels of phytoandrogens.

Pine pollen may be more effective when applied externally, especially for people with digestive issues.

Pine pollen should be used in moderation to prevent excess testosterone and resulting estrogen overload.

Pine pollen should be cycled — 3 weeks on and 1 week off, or 2 weeks on 2 weeks off — or used irregularly (1-2 times/week).

PINE POLLEN USES

- Longevity, antiaging, regeneration, and rejuvenation
- Vitality, energy, spirit, and stamina
- Sexual and reproductive function
- Rest and recovery support, athletic and otherwise
- Cardiovascular health
- Neuroprotective and neuroregenerative
- Connective tissue strengthening
- Stress management (adrenal/thyroid health)
- Immune system support
- Blood sugar balance
- Detoxification (liver, kidney, lymph tissues)
- Weight management
- Pain alleviation
- Antioxidant, anti-cancer, and anti-inflammatory

Pine pollen contains phytosterols, amino acids, vitamin A, beta carotene, B vitamins, vitamin C, vitamin D, vitamin E, essential fatty acids, flavonoids, polyphenols, MSM (methylsulfonylmethane), SOD (superoxide dismutase), pycnogenol, resveratrol, quercetin, glutathione, magnesium, calcium, manganese, selenium, zinc, copper, and iron.

Pine pollen can be consumed in powder form, as a tea, capsule, tincture, infusion, or extract.

Traditional preparation: varies; sold as powdered extract.

The Natural Path to Hormonal Wellness, Part 1 by Katarina Nolte
Pages: 201 (23,609 words); Copyright © 2014 by Katarina Nolte.
All rights reserved. http://katarinanolte.com/ July 2014

NOTE

Do not consume with sugar or sweeteners. Sugar and sweeteners are counter effective to hormonal balance.

LEARN MORE

The Natural Testosterone Plan: For Sexual Health and Energy - Stephen Harrod Buhner - Google Books
http://goo.gl/AAhL3C
Phytoandrogens - Wikipedia, the free encyclopedia
http://en.wikipedia.org/wiki/Phytoandrogens
Novel phytoandrogens and lipidic a ugmenters from Eucommia ulmoides. [BMC Complement Altern Med. 2007] - PubMed - NCBI
http://www.ncbi.nlm.nih.gov/pubmed/17261169
HEALTH AND THE ENVIRONMENT: Testosterone Levels Fall Worldwide | Global Research
http://www.globalresearch.ca/health-and-the-environment-testosterone-levels-fall-worldwide/30129
Pine Pollen - Boost testosterone and balance hormones | Natural News
http://www.naturalnews.com/031867_pine_pollen_testosterone.html#
How Do I Restore Testosterone Levels? | LIVESTRONG.COM
http://www.livestrong.com/article/248499-how-do-i-restore-testosterone-levels/
Phytoandrogens - Wikipedia, the free encyclopedia
http://en.wikipedia.org/wiki/Phytoandrogens
Phytosterol - Wikipedia, the free encyclopedia
http://en.wikipedia.org/wiki/Phytosterol
Androgen Testosterone » Herbs Male Enhancement
http://androgentestosterone.com/herbs-male-enhancement

The Natural Path to Hormonal Wellness, Part 1 by Katarina Nolte
Pages: 201 (23,609 words); Copyright © 2014 by Katarina Nolte.
All rights reserved. http://katarinanolte.com/ July 2014

Pine Pollen - Serendipity Superfoods
http://www.serendipitysuperfoods.com/pine-pollen.html
Pinus massoniana - Wikipedia, the free encyclopedia
http://en.wikipedia.org/wiki/Pinus_massoniana
Raw Pine Pollen & Phyto-androgens at The Truth in Medicine, topic 1744232 | Cure Zone
http://curezone.org/forums/am.asp?i=1744232
How To Make Poultices And Compresses | Whispering Earth
http://whisperingearth.co.uk/2011/08/23/how-to-make-poultices-and-compresses/
Pine Pollen Tea | Green world Natural herbal & Organic supplements Online
http://shop.nutrition-sa.com/products/pine-pollen-tea
Using Pure Pine Pollen for Tincturing - Pine Pollen | RAW Forest Foods
http://www.rawforestfoodsblog.com/using-pure-pine-pollen-for-tincturing/
Steroids: Herbal Anabolic | Free Fitness Guru
http://www.freefitnessguru.com/blog/tag/steroids-herbal-anabolic

Different herbs work in different ways to increase androgen levels in the body.
The Royal Androgenic Herb: Pine Pollen | RAW Forest Foods
http://www.rawforestfoodsblog.com/the-royal-androgenic-herb-pine-pollen/

The Natural Path to Hormonal Wellness, Part 1 by Katarina Nolte
Pages: 201 (23,609 words); Copyright © 2014 by Katarina Nolte.
All rights reserved. http://katarinanolte.com/ July 2014

SARSAPARILLA

One person who was keenly aware of plant saponins was Russell Marker, a maverick biochemist. In 1939 he published a study on sarsasapogenin, the saponin in Smilax used to make sarsaparilla. The next year he published studies on diosgenin, a saponin isolated from a Mexican yam species of the genus Dioscorea. From diosgenin he was able to synthesize the human hormone testosterone in eight steps and progesterone in just five steps.
MEXICAN YAMS | UCLA Mildred E. Mathias Botanical Garden
http://www.botgard.ucla.edu/html/botanytextbooks/economicbotany/Dioscoreamed/

Sarsaparilla (smilax) is native to Central America and has traditionally been used in the Caribbean, China, India, and Europe for the treatment of infections and female problems.

Sarsaparilla possesses adaptogenic and stimulant properties. Among other things, it is said to stimulate progesterone production.

The popular TCM (Traditional Chinese Medicine) herbal blend known as myomin contains sarsaparilla. Myomin is used as a natural aromatase inhibitor, meant to prevent testosterone from converting into estrogen, as well as a xenoestrogen detoxifier, helping the body rid itself of artificial estrogen-like substances.

106

The Natural Path to Hormonal Wellness, Part 1 by Katarina Nolte
Pages: 201 (23,609 words); Copyright © 2014 by Katarina Nolte.
All rights reserved. http://katarinanolte.com/ July 2014

Sarsaparilla should be cycled — 3 weeks on and 1 week off, or 2 weeks on 2 weeks off — or used irregularly (1-2 times/week).

SARSAPARILLA USES

- Connective tissue strengthening
- Sexual and reproductive function
- Rest and recovery support, athletic and otherwise
- Detoxification (liver, kidney, lymph tissues)
- Gastrointestinal health
- Pain alleviation
- Immune system support
- Antibacterial, antifungal, antiviral, antioxidant, and anti-inflammatory

Sarsaparilla contains beta sitosterol, stigmasterol, saponins, vitamin A, vitamin D, manganese, zinc, and iron.

Sarsaparilla can be consumed in powder form, as a tea, capsule, spice, tincture, infusion, or extract.

Traditional preparation: decoction, tincture.

NOTE

Do not consume with sugar or sweeteners. Sugar and sweeteners are counter effective to hormonal balance.

The Natural Path to Hormonal Wellness, Part 1 by Katarina Nolte
Pages: 201 (23,609 words); Copyright © 2014 by Katarina Nolte.
All rights reserved. http://katarinanolte.com/ July 2014

LEARN MORE

Sarsaparilla (soft drink) - Wikipedia, the free encyclopedia
http://en.wikipedia.org/wiki/Sarsaparilla_(soft_drink)
Smilax regelii - Wikipedia, the free encyclopedia
http://en.wikipedia.org/wiki/Smilax_regelii
Tropical Plant Database entry for: Sarsaparilla (Smilax officinalis) (Smilax aristolochiaefolia) (Smilax glabra) (Smilax febrifuga) (Smilx ornata) | Rain Tree
http://www.rain-tree.com/sarsaparilla.htm#.Ukq-q9LIA2c
25 Best Ways to Detox From Heavy Metals, Pesticides, Environmental Pollutants, and Metabolic Waste - Waking Times
http://www.wakingtimes.com/2013/07/18/25-best-ways-to-detox-from-heavy-metals-pesticides-environmental-pollutants-and-metabolic-waste/
Natural Body Cleansing and Toxin Removal | Healing Edge
http://www.healingedge.net/store/article_detoxification.html
Aromatase Inhibitors - Learn about Aromatase Inhibitors | MP Research Supply
http://www.mpresearchsupply.com/store/pages.php?pageid=17
John Gray explains how Myomin helps balance estrogen hormone levels - YouTube
http://youtu.be/QmwzMs3RinU
Sarsaparilla - Medicinal Herb Info
http://medicinalherbinfo.org/herbs/Sarsaparilla.html

Postmenopausal women say oatstraw turns a vaginal desert into a flowing oasis.
Sexy Herbs by Susun S. Weed | Wisdom Magazine
http://wisdom-magazine.com/Article.aspx/2431/

The Natural Path to Hormonal Wellness, Part 1 by Katarina Nolte
Pages: 201 (23,609 words); Copyright © 2014 by Katarina Nolte.
All rights reserved. http://katarinanolte.com/ July 2014

SCHIZANDRA

*Even younger women, including those in their teens
and 20s, can suffer from estrogen dominance. Their
symptoms may include PMS, weight gain, fibrocystic
breasts, bloating, troublesome periods, infertility,
endometriosis, depression or repeated miscarriage.*
**LE Magazine, June 2003 - Report: The Overlooked
Female Hormone**
http://www.lef.org/magazine/mag2003/jun2003_repor
t_female_01.htm

Schizandra is native to Eastern Asia and is one of
the herbs used in TCM (traditional Chinese
medicine). Schizandra has traditionally been used
as an immune booster and for the treatment of
female problems by various Asian peoples.

Schizandra possesses adaptogenic properties.

Schizandra may have to be cycled.

SCHIZANDRA USES

- Vitality, energy, spirit, and stamina
- Immune system support
- Detoxification (liver, kidney, lymph tissues)
- Neuroprotective and neuroregenerative
- Cardiovascular health
- Respiratory health
- Sexual and reproductive function
- Rest and recovery support, athletic and otherwise
- Stress management (adrenal/thyroid health)

109

- Longevity, antiaging, regeneration, and rejuvenation
- Connective tissue strengthening
- Pain alleviation
- Gastrointestinal health
- Blood sugar balance
- Anti-inflammatory, antioxidant, and antiviral

Schizandra contains polyphenols, stigmasterol, beta sitosterol, vitamin A, vitamin C, magnesium, and chromium.

The medicinal schizandra berries and seeds can be consumed whole, in powder form, as a tea, capsule, spice, tincture, infusion, or extract.

Traditional preparation: tea, tincture.

NOTE

Do not consume with sugar or sweeteners. Sugar and sweeteners are counter effective to hormonal balance.

LEARN MORE

Schisandra chinensis - Wikipedia, the free encyclopedia
http://en.wikipedia.org/wiki/Schisandra_chinensis
Down There: Sexual and Reproductive Health the Wise Woman Way (Wise Woman Herbal Series) by Susun S. Weed
http://www.amazon.com/Down-There-Sexual-Reproductive-Health/dp/1888123133

Chinese medicine: Schizandra berry a potent adaptogenic herb | Natural News
http://www.naturalnews.com/009229_schizandra_schisandra.html

How to Grow Schisandra | Home Guides | SF Gate
http://homeguides.sfgate.com/grow-schisandra-21534.html

Herbal Medicine: 50 Fundamental Herbs | Nature Antidote
http://natureantidote.blogspot.com/2009/09/50-fundamental-herbs.html

Ron Teeguarden - Goji & Schizandra Drops
http://www.yahwehsaliveandwell.com/item_39/Goji-Schizandra-Drops.htm

Schisandra for a Healthier Erection | Herballove.com
http://www.herballove.com/solutions/schisandra-healthier-erection

Traditional Chinese Medicine/TCM and Menopause | TCM Page
http://www.tcmpage.com/hpmenopause.html

Health Benefits of Chinese Herb Schizandra - Where to Buy Schisandra Fruit Online | SONI 2006
http://soni2006.hubpages.com/hub/Health-Benefits-of-Chinese-Herb-Schizandra-Where-to-Buy-Schisandra-Fruit

Beta sitosterol prevents aromatase from converting testosterone to estradiol, preserving the integrity of the testosterone your body makes.
Endosterol for Healthy Prostate and Abundant Testosterone | Peak Health Now
http://www.peak-health-now.com/endosterol-prostate-testosterone.html

SUMA

My grandmother followed her gynecologist's advice to the letter, developed breast cancer and died.
Is Maca better at Balance Hormones than Progesterone?
http://www.healthguidance.org/entry/1679/1/Is-Maca-better-at-Balance-Hormones-than-Progesterone.html

Suma is an adaptogenic plant native to South America. It is known as the 'Brazilian ginseng' and as such has traditionally been used to treat anything and everything.

Suma root has stimulant properties.

Suma should be cycled — 3 weeks on and 1 week off, or 2 weeks on 2 weeks off — or used irregularly (1-2 times/week).

SUMA USES

- Stress management (adrenal/thyroid health)
- Pain alleviation
- Immune system support
- Sexual and reproductive function
- Vitality, energy, spirit, and stamina
- Respiratory health
- Cardiovascular health
- Longevity, antiaging, regeneration, and rejuvenation
- Blood sugar balance

- Neuroprotective and neuroregenerative
- Connective tissue strengthening
- Rest and recovery support, athletic and otherwise
- Gastrointestinal health
- Detoxification
- Weight management
- Anti-inflammatory, anti-allergy, anti-ulcer, antibacterial, antiviral, anti-cancer, antifungal, and anti-tumor

Suma contains saponins, beta sitosterol, stigmasterol, amino acids, vitamin A, B vitamins, vitamin E, vitamin K, germanium, magnesium, zinc, and iron.

The medicinal suma root can be consumed whole, in powder form, as a tea, capsule, spice, tincture, infusion, or extract.

Traditional preparation: decoction.

NOTE

Do not consume with sugar or sweeteners. Sugar and sweeteners are counter effective to hormonal balance.

LEARN MORE

Hebanthe eriantha - Wikipedia, the free encyclopedia
http://en.wikipedia.org/wiki/Hebanthe_eriantha

Tropical Plant Database entry for: Suma (Pfaffia paniculata) (Pfaffia glomerata) | Rain Tree
http://www.rain-tree.com/suma.htm#.U5OrBnJdWSo

Suma Root Medicinal Uses Benefits | Annie's Remedy
http://www.anniesremedy.com/herb_detail508.php

SuperOrganicFoods: Premium Suma Root Powder
https://www.superorganicfoods.com/product_info.php?products_id=160

What is Suma? - Global Healing Center
http://www.globalhealingcenter.com/natural-health/what-is-suma/

Suma Testosterone Root » The Amazonian Ecdysterone « Hebanthe Eriantha | Anabolic Men
http://anabolicmen.com/suma-testosterone-root/

Jack up your testosterone - Paleohacks
http://paleohacks.com/questions/29354/jack-up-your-testosterone.html

"Norms" Aren't So Normal: The normal level of testosterone has been reduced by the medical community as well. They simply decided to make a new norm since everyone's testosterone levels are lower than they were 50 years ago.

T NATION | Fight the T-Killing Toxins
http://www.t-nation.com/free_online_article/most_recent/fight_the_t_killing_toxins

The Natural Path to Hormonal Wellness, Part 1 by Katarina Nolte
Pages: 201 (23,609 words); Copyright © 2014 by Katarina Nolte.
All rights reserved. http://katarinanolte.com/ July 2014

TRIBULUS

Increasing testosterone in the blood can restore health and reverse the signs of aging, thereby reducing many of the side effects, for mood, memory and heart health.

Herbs and Vitamins can Increase Testosterone | Natural News

http://www.naturalnews.com/026832_testosterone_herbs_vitamins.html#

Tribulus terrestris (puncturevine) is native to South Asia. Tribulus has adaptogenic properties, is part of TCM (traditional Chinese medicine) and the Indian Ayurvedic medicine and has traditionally been used as an aphrodisiac and for female problems.

Tribulus terrestris may cause a rise in progesterone levels, which in some cases may lead to proportionately lower estrogen/xenoestrogen levels and resultingly higher testosterone levels.

Tribulus alatus, a desert version of the tribulus plant, may increase androgen levels by reducing cortisol and stimulate anabolism.

Quality can be of concern when it comes to the effectiveness of tribulus terrestris. One should opt for pesticide free, organic, wild harvested tribulus.

Tribulus should be cycled — 3 weeks on and 1 week off, or 2 weeks on 2 weeks off — or used irregularly (1-2 times/week).

115

TRIBULUS TERRESTRIS USES

- Connective tissue strengthening
- Longevity, antiaging, regeneration, and rejuvenation
- Sexual and reproductive function
- Rest and recovery support, athletic and otherwise
- Cardiovascular health
- Detoxification
- Stress management
- Gastrointestinal health
- Cardiovascular health
- Anti-inflammatory, antibacterial, antiviral, and antioxidant

Tribulus terrestris contains beta sitosterol, saponins, tannins, alkaloids, and bioflavonoids.

Tribulus can be consumed in powder form, as a tea, capsule, tincture, infusion, or extract.

Traditional preparation: N/A.

NOTE

Do not consume with sugar or sweeteners. Sugar and sweeteners are counter effective to hormonal balance.

LEARN MORE

Tribulus terrestris - Wikipedia, the free encyclopedia
http://en.wikipedia.org/wiki/Tribulus_terrestris

116

5 Coolest Benefits of Tribulus Terrestris – Widgets WP
http://widgets.wp.com/likes/#blog_id=7002972&post_id=3&origin=dbrawlmuscle.wordpress.com&obj_id=7002972-3-5249943d4a89a

Tribulus Terrestris Medicinal Uses – Annie's Remedy
http://www.anniesremedy.com/herb_detail250.php

Beyond Tribulus: the Truth Uncovered! | Anabolic Extreme
http://www.anabolicextreme.com/archives/anex_archives_issue13_tribulus.htm

Dioscin, a natural steroid saponin, shows remarkable protective effect against acetaminophen-induced liver damage in vitro and in vivo. [Toxicol Lett. 2012] - PubMed - NCBI
http://www.ncbi.nlm.nih.gov/pubmed/22939915

What Is Steroidal Saponins? | eHow
http://www.ehow.com/facts_5525189_steroidal-saponins.html

Diosgenin - Wikipedia, the free encyclopedia
http://en.wikipedia.org/wiki/Diosgenin

Dioscin, Protodioscin, Gracillin, Protogracillin, Diosgenin - Bioknow Science and Technology Co. Ltd
http://xuanning.en.ec21.com/Dioscin_Protodioscin_Gracillin_Protogracillin_Diosgenin--1094125_1094181.html

The Effect of Oral Feeding of Tribulus terrestris L. on Sex Hormone and Gonadotropin Levels in Addicted Male Rats | ncbi.nlm.nih.gov
http://www.ncbi.nlm.nih.gov/pmc/articles/PMC3850326/

Tribulus Terrestris Benefits – CurEase | High Dose Resveratrol Acai
http://highdoseresveratrolacai.com/product_info.php?products_id=65

Tribulus components don't convert to testosterone | Ergo Log
http://www.ergo-log.com/tribulusdoping.html

Not Tribulus terrestris, but Tribulus alatus | Ergo Log
http://www.ergo-log.com/tribulusalatus.html

Free serum testosterone level in male rats treated with Tribulus alatus extracts. [Int Braz J Urol. 2007 Jul-Aug] - PubMed - NCBI
http://www.ncbi.nlm.nih.gov/pubmed/17767762

What is Tribulus Alatus or T-Alatus? | Prohormones Direct
http://prohormonesdirect.com/what-is-tribulus-alatus-or-t-alatus/

Hv, Question about Tribulus and natural AI at The Truth in Medicine, topic 1827368 | Cure Zone
http://curezone.org/forums/am.asp?i=1827368

Herbs That Increase Testosterone Levels | LIVESTRONG.COM
http://www.livestrong.com/article/70578-herbs-increase-testosterone-levels/

Adrenal exhaustion. Symptoms, causes, tests, remedies | Grow Youthful
http://www.growyouthful.com/ailment/adrenal-exhaustion.php

Fatigue solution natural supplements and vitamins | Tribulus Terrestris Extract
http://www.tribulusterrestrisextract.com/fatigue.html

Adaptogens for Adrenal Fatigue | EI Resources
http://www.ei-resource.org/community/groups/viewdiscussion/58-adaptogens-adaptogens-for-adrenal-fatigue?groupid=8

List of natural adaptogens | Plantae | Adaptogens
http://adaptogens.com/plantae/

Herbal Hormone Balance | Herbal Aromatase Inhibitor | Harmony | New Vita
http://www.newvita.com/shopdisplayproducts.asp?catalogid=103

Buyer's Guide: The Best Testosterone Products - Nutrition Express Articles
http://www.nutritionexpress.com/showarticle.aspx?articleid=781
Can You Grow Muscle From Anabolic Plants? | Iron Man Magazine
www.ironmanmagazine.com/can-you-grow-muscle-from-anabolic-plants/

Testosterone strengthens the heart muscle; there are more testosterone receptors in the heart than in any other muscle. Testosterone lowers LDL cholesterol and total cholesterol and improves every cardiac risk factor. It has been shown to improve or eliminate arrhythmia and angina. Testosterone replacement is the most underutilized important treatment for heart disease.
Testosterone Therapy & HGH Therapy | Atlantic Rejuvenation
http://atlanticrejuvenation.com/testosterone-therapy.html

VITEX

Every herb will react differently for each person.
**Herbal Infertility Treatments | Herbs to Get
Pregnant | Natural Fertility Info**
http://natural-fertility-info.com/fertility-herbs-fertility-supplements.html

Vitex (chastetree) is native to the Mediterranean region and has adaptogenic properties. Vitex has traditionally been used for female problems.

Vitex may cause a rise in progesterone levels, which in some cases may lead to proportionately lower estrogen/xenoestrogen levels and resultingly higher testosterone levels.

Vitex may also stimulate a rise in LH (luteinizing hormone) and a reduction in prolactin levels, both of which are associated with higher levels of free (bioavailable) testosterone.

Vitex may not have to be cycled.

VITEX USES

- Sexual and reproductive function
- Connective tissue strengthening
- Edema prevention
- Stress management
- Anti-cancer and anti-tumor

120

Vitex contains phytosterols and bioflavonoids.

Vitex can be consumed in powder form, as a tea, capsule, tincture, infusion, or extract.

Traditional preparation: tincture.

NOTE

Do not consume with sugar or sweeteners. Sugar and sweeteners are counter effective to hormonal balance.

LEARN MORE

Xenohormones and xenoestrogens - Women Living Naturally
http://www.womenlivingnaturally.com/articlepage.php?id=73
Chaste Tree Berry Fertility Dosage Medicinal Uses Benefits | Annie's Remedy
http://www.anniesremedy.com/herb_detail213.php
Vitex Tincture For PMS | Annie's Remedy
http://www.anniesremedy.com/chart_remedy.php?remID=266
Painful Menses Tea | Annie's Remedy
http://www.anniesremedy.com/chart_remedy.php?remID=158
Endocrine Tonic For Menopause | Annie's Remedy
http://www.anniesremedy.com/chart_remedy.php?remID=198
Estrogen Dominance|Women Living Naturally
http://www.womenlivingnaturally.com/articlepage.php?id=72

Women Suffer Needlessly from Confusion about Hormones | Natural News
http://www.naturalnews.com/025812_hormones_drug_estrogen.html

Better Nutrition Magazine: Supplements, Nutrition, Recipes, Personal Care – Ask the Naturopath
http://www.betternutrition.com/xenoestrogensenvironmentalhormones/columns/askthenaturopath/698

An Update on Plant Derived Anti-Androgens — International Journal of Endocrinology and Metabolism | Kowsar
http://endometabol.com/?page=article&article_id=3644

Natural Hormone Optimization Made Simple & Cheap: Avoid These 10 Anti-Androgens to Boost Testosterone & DHT - SuppVersity
http://suppversity.blogspot.com/2012/05/natural-hormone-optimization-made.html

ANTIFUNGAL ACTIVITIES OF VITEX NEGUNDO LINN
http://www.pakbs.org/pjbot/PDFs/41(4)/PJB41(4)1941.pdf

Vitex - Chasteberry - Monk's Pepper - Vitex Negundo - Vitex Agnus Castus | Herbs Guide
http://www.herbsguide.net/vitex.html

Natural Progesterone Herbs | LIVESTRONG.COM
http://www.livestrong.com/article/445374-natural-progesterone-herbs/

Vitex agnus-castus - Wikipedia, the free encyclopedia
http://en.wikipedia.org/wiki/Vitex_agnus-castus#Herbal_uses

Vitex - What Should You Know About It?
http://altmedicine.about.com/od/herbsupplementguide/a/Vitex.htm

Herb Profile: Vitex or Chaste Tree - Wellness Mama
http://wellnessmama.com/8314/herb-profile-vitex/

The Natural Path to Hormonal Wellness, Part 1 by Katarina Nolte
Pages: 201 (23,609 words); Copyright © 2014 by Katarina Nolte.
All rights reserved. http://katarinanolte.com/ July 2014

TESTOSTERONE NATION | Vitex - Page 1

http://tnation.t-nation.com/free_online_forum/sports_body_training_performance_bodybuilding/vitex

Environmental impact of pharmaceuticals and personal care products - Wikipedia, the free encyclopedia

http://en.wikipedia.org/wiki/Environmental_impact_of_pharmaceuticals_and_personal_care_products

NOAA - National Oceanic and Atmospheric Administration - Protecting Lives & Property

http://www.noaa.gov/features/protecting_1208/pharmaceuticals.html

Streams stressed by pharmaceutical pollution | Cary Institute of Ecosystem Studies

http://www.caryinstitute.org/newsroom/streams-stressed-pharmaceutical-pollution

Pharmaceutical pollution damages ecosystems, U.S. study shows - World Israel News | Haaretz

http://www.haaretz.com/news/world/pharmaceutical-pollution-damages-ecosystems-u-s-study-shows.premium-1.514488

Pharmaceuticals and Personal Care Products (PPCPs) | US EPA

http://www.epa.gov/ppcp/

What Increases Progesterone & Estrogen? | LIVESTRONG.COM

http://www.livestrong.com/article/336927-what-increases-progesterone-estrogen/

Ayurvedic Herbs for the Pituitary Gland | LIVESTRONG.COM

http://www.livestrong.com/article/149355-ayurvedic-herbs-for-the-pituitary-gland/

On the other hand women lacking Testosterone suffer from a general lack of libido and experience difficulty achieving orgasm. This condition can be treated with the supplementation of a low-dose Testosterone as a topical cream; can be used successfully and without side effects. Testosterone can recapture the natural balance of hormones that one enjoyed when at the physical and mental peaks; it will enhance sex drive, relieve menopausal symptoms; restores energy, and strengthens bone and relieves depression.

Testosterone pellets treat adrenal fatigue - Dr. Dalal Akoury

http://www.awaremed.com/testosterone-pellets-treat-adrenal-fatigue/

The Natural Path to Hormonal Wellness, Part 1 by Katarina Nolte
Pages: 201 (23,609 words); Copyright © 2014 by Katarina Nolte.
All rights reserved. http://katarinanolte.com/ July 2014

WILD YAM

At the practice we have learned that most women don't understand that unhappiness is a form of stress.
Estrogen Dominance - Is It Real? | Women to Women
http://www.womentowomen.com/hormonal-imbalance/estrogen-dominance/

Wild yam (dioscorea villosa) is native to Central and South America and is one of the many herbs used in TCM (traditional Chinese medicine).

Wild yam has traditionally been used for female problems.

Wild yam has adaptogenic properties.

Opinions on wild yam in relation to hormonal reactions in the human body vary. Some believe that wild yam stimulates the body's production of progesterone levels. Others believe that wild yam leads to an increased production of estrogen which would require an increase in the body's production of testosterone. There are also those who believe that wild yam has an effect comparable to that of DHEA (dehydroepiandrosterone).

Wild yam should be cycled —2 weeks on 2 weeks off — or used irregularly (1-2 times/week).

125

The Natural Path to Hormonal Wellness, Part 1 by Katarina Nolte
Pages: 201 (23,609 words); Copyright © 2014 by Katarina Nolte.
All rights reserved. http://katarinanolte.com/ July 2014

WILD YAM USES

- Sexual and reproductive function
- Cardiovascular health
- Respiratory health
- Gastrointestinal health
- Connective tissue strengthening
- Pain alleviation
- Stress management (adrenal/thyroid health)
- Neuroprotective and neuroregenerative
- Antioxidant, anti-inflammatory, antiviral, antifungal, anti-cancer, and anti-tumor

Wild yam contains phytosterols, saponins, alkaloids, tannins, B vitamins, beta carotene, vitamin C, magnesium, chromium, selenium, and zinc.

The medicinal wild yam root can be consumed in powder form, capsule, as a tea, or extract.

Traditional preparation: tea, tincture.

NOTE

Do not consume with sugar or sweeteners. Sugar and sweeteners are counter effective to hormonal balance.

LEARN MORE

Wild Yam Root Medicinal Uses Benefits | Annie's Remedy
http://www.anniesremedy.com/herb_detail119.php

126

The Natural Path to Hormonal Wellness, Part 1 by Katarina Nolte
Pages: 201 (23,609 words); Copyright © 2014 by Katarina Nolte.
All rights reserved. http://katarinanolte.com/ July 2014

Table of Adaptogenic Herbs Used to Treat Adrenal Gland Dysfunction | The Association for the Advancement of Restorative Medicine
http://restorativemedicine.org/books/fundamentals-of-naturopathic-endocrinology/professionals/adrenal-metabolism-disorders/table-of-adaptogenic-herbs-used-to-treat-adrenal-gland-dysfunction/

Wild Yam Extract – Mountain Rose Herbs
https://www.mountainroseherbs.com/products/wild-yam-extract/profile

Menopause, HRT, and Nutrition - Nutri-Notes Newsletter Vol 3, #6
http://www.nutri-notes.com/novdec96_simple.htm

The study further states that natural progesterone secretion suppresses oestradiol receptors in both the endometrium and breast tissue, and has an anti-oestrogen effect (just as, for example, the latest aromatase inhibitors aim to do), but that very high concentrations of synthetic progestins can stimulate human breast cancer cells.

Healing Pastures » Natural Aromatase Inhibitors
http://healingpastures.com/2009/10/18/natural-aromatase-inhibitors/

The Natural Path to Hormonal Wellness, Part 1 by Katarina Nolte
Pages: 201 (23,609 words); Copyright © 2014 by Katarina Nolte.
All rights reserved. http://katarinanolte.com/ July 2014

YOHIMBE

The average American eats 14 pounds of chemicals each year—2 pounds of these are pesticides and herbicides.
FACT LIBRARY | Just Do One
http://www.justdoone.org/videocontest/facts

Yohimbe is a tree native to West Africa belonging to the coffee family.

Yohimbe has traditionally been used for its aphrodisiac and stimulant properties.

Yohimbe may cause side effects related to its stimulant properties. These may be avoided by limiting the consumption to topical applications.

Yohimbe should not be consumed on a regular basis.

YOHIMBE USES

- Sexual and reproductive function
- Weight management
- Stress management
- Vitality, energy, spirit, and stamina

Yohimbe contains alkaloids, tannins, and yohimbine (active chemical).

Yohimbe can be consumed in powder form, capsule, as a tea, decoction, or extract.

Traditional preparation: tea, tincture.

NOTE

Do not consume with sugar or sweeteners. Sugar and sweeteners are counter effective to hormonal balance.

LEARN MORE

Yohimbine - Wikipedia, the free encyclopedia
http://en.wikipedia.org/wiki/Yohimbine
Rubiaceae - Wikipedia, the free encyclopedia
http://en.wikipedia.org/wiki/Rubiaceae
**Yohimbe Bark Extract Medicinal Uses Benefits |
Annie's Remedy**
http://www.anniesremedy.com/herb_detail295.php
Yohimbe Bark Tea | Annie's Remedy
http://www.anniesremedy.com/chart_remedy.php?rem
_ID=457

*Alcohol, fattening, stress, illness, statins,
serotoninergics & all diseases & trauma suppress
androgens.*
**THE NEED FOR TESTOSTERONE AS PART OF
BIOIDENTICAL HRT BHT FOR MEN & WOMEN**
http://www.compounding.co.za/howtoprescribebiohor
mones.htm

NUTRIENTS

ASTAXANTHIN

Astaxanthin belongs to a class of naturally-occurring pigments called carotenoids.
Astaxanthin | Antioxidant Supplement - Mercola.com
http://products.mercola.com/astaxanthin/

Astaxanthin is a fat soluble antioxidant in the carotenoid family, found in bell peppers, red beets, wild fish and seafood, and seaweeds (algae).

Because it is fat soluble it should be consumed with healthy fats for optimal absorption. Astaxanthin may be incompatible with vitamin E and should therefore not be consumed at the same time.

ASTAXANTHIN USES

- Stress management
- Cellular protection
- Neuroprotective and neuroregenerative
- Vitality, energy, and stamina
- Connective tissue strengthening
- Rest and recovery support, athletic and otherwise
- Immune system support

The Natural Path to Hormonal Wellness, Part 1 by Katarina Nolte
Pages: 201 (23,609 words); Copyright © 2014 by Katarina Nolte.
All rights reserved. http://katarinanolte.com/ July 2014

- Longevity, antiaging, regeneration, and rejuvenation
- Sexual and reproductive function
- Gastrointestinal health
- Cardiovascular health
- Weight management
- Detoxification
- Anti-inflammatory, antioxidant, anti-cancer, and antibacterial

The best sources of astaxanthin are the aforementioned whole foods, seaweeds and supplemental microalgae (phytoplankton) powders or capsules.

Sources of industrial astaxanthin like those found in farmed fish and farmed seafood, as well as petrochemical- or fungus-based astaxanthin supplements should be avoided.

NOTE

Do not consume with sugar or sweeteners. Sugar and sweeteners are counter effective to hormonal balance.

LEARN MORE

Astaxanthin - Wikipedia, the free encyclopedia
http://en.wikipedia.org/wiki/Astaxanthin
Astaxanthin Health Benefits - Prostate.net
http://www.prostate.net/prostate-health-supplements-a-z/astaxanthin-health-benefits/

**Astaxanthin supplement raises testosterone level |
Ergo Log**
http://www.ergo-
log.com/astaxanthinetestosterone.html
**The Antioxidant Astaxanthin: An Interview with
Rudi Moerck | Articles | Mercola**
http://articles.mercola.com/sites/articles/archive/201
1/12/11/rudi-moerck-on-astaxanthin.aspx
**Astaxanthin: A Review of the Literature - Natural
Medicine Journal: The Official Journal of the
American Association of Naturopathic Physicians**
http://www.naturalmedicinejournal.com/article_conte
nt.asp?article=293
**Update Astaxantin DHT and Hairloss | Hair Loss
Research**
http://www.hairloss-
research.org/UpdateAstaxantinDHT4-12.html

*These antioxidants protect against breast cancer,
prostate cancer, and stomach cancer, due to their
high carotenoid content.*
**NYC Personal Trainer teaches how to Get Rid fat
With Greens | Best gym in Brooklyn**
http://krankbrooklyn.com/blog/get-rid-of-the-belly-
with-greens/

CALCIUM D-GLUCARATE

Results indicated that enhancing progesterone decreased testosterone. Such results raise concerns because testosterone plays an important role in tissue growth. Progesterone-induced testosterone suppression could, therefore, lead to wasting and injury.

Side Effects Of Micronized Natural Progesterone | LIVESTRONG.COM

http://www.livestrong.com/article/315126-side-effects-of-micronized-natural-progesterone/

Calcium D-glucarate is the supplemental form of glucaric acid.

Glucaric acid is a nutrient found in cruciferous vegetables, beans, peas, sprouts, melons, lettuce, tomatoes, peppers, cucumbers, apples, apricots, berries, cherries, and citrus fruits.

CALCIUM D-GLUCARATE USES

- Detoxification (liver, kidney, lymph tissues)
- Sexual and reproductive function
- Antioxidant, anti-cancer, and anti-tumor

The main benefit of consuming calcium D-glucarate supplements and foods containing glucaric acid is xenoestrogen removal.

Hormonal balance and a proportionate increase in testosterone can only occur if we consistently work on eliminating xenoestrogenic substances like pesticides, herbicides, insecticides, chlorine and other industrial toxins from our bodies.

NOTE

Do not consume with sugar or sweeteners. Sugar and sweeteners are counter effective to hormonal balance.

LEARN MORE

Foods High in Glucaric Acid | LIVESTRONG.COM
http://www.livestrong.com/article/330279-foods-high-in-glucaric-acid/
What Foods Provide Calcium D-glucarate? | LIVESTRONG.COM
http://www.livestrong.com/article/30822-foods-provide-calcium-dglucarate/
Health Benefits of Calcium D-Glucarate for Clearing Xenoestrogens - OMTimes Writer's Community
http://community.omtimes.com/profiles/blogs/health-benefits-of-calcium-d-glucarate-for-clearing-xenoestrogens
Uzo Onukwugha - EzineArticles.com Expert Author
http://ezinearticles.com/?expert=Uzo_Onukwugha
Holistic approach for estrogen dominance, breast cancer awareness - Ahwatukee Foothills News: Community Focus
http://www.ahwatukee.com/community_focus/article_30f53a00-0cc3-11e2-bb9b-001a4bcf887a.html
Best aromatase inhibitor supplement - Bodybuilding.com Forums
http://forum.bodybuilding.com/showthread.php?t=116999991

The Natural Path to Hormonal Wellness, Part 1 by Katarina Nolte
Pages: 201 (23,609 words); Copyright © 2014 by Katarina Nolte.
All rights reserved. http://katarinanolte.com/ July 2014

Estrogen Dominance - The Bane of Infertility Issues - Both Male and Female Fertility | Ezine Articles
http://ezinearticles.com/?Estrogen-Dominance---The-Bane-of-Infertility-Issues---Both-Male-and-Female-Fertility&id=3047088
Naked Truth: Xenoestrogens | T NATION
http://www.t-nation.com/free_online_article/sports_body_training_performance_interviews/naked_truth_xenoestrogens;jsessionid=230D5920B55E9083F2D327A94648265D-mcd02.hydra

Raw, cruciferous vegetables are natural thyroid depressants because they contain isothiocyanates, which naturally interfere with the hormone production of the thyroid. Not long ago we featured an article, Why You Need to Cook These Vegetables for Maximum Nutrition, that encouraged readers to cook cruciferous vegetables like broccoli, collards, cabbage and kale because when eaten raw, these vegetables suppress the thyroid. If you currently suffer from hypothyroidism (under-active thyroid), these veggies will suppress your thyroid function and slow down your metabolism even further.

Natural Factors that Suppress Your Hormone Production - and How to Avoid Them | Body Ecology
http://bodyecology.com/articles/suppress_hormone_production.php#.UKIeFOQ8CSo

CHRYSIN

In reality, women may develop symptoms of androgen deficiency at any age, from their teen years through late adulthood.
Testosterone insufficiency in women: fact or fiction? » Sexual Medicine » BUMC
http://www.bumc.bu.edu/sexualmedicine/publications/testosterone-insufficiency-in-women-fact-or-fiction/

Chrysin is a bioflavonoid found in passion fruit, whole raw honey (honey, propolis, bee pollen and honeycomb), and in the Ayurvedic herb known as the Indian trumpet flower.

Peppers contain a nutrient called piperine, which, when consumed with chrysin, improves its absorption of chrysin. This may explain the fact that in Mexico passion fruit is traditionally consumed with chili powder and lime.

Hot peppers, by the way, tend to increase the absorption of all nutrients, including those found in herbs and supplements.

CHRYSIN USES

- Sexual and reproductive function
- Stress management (adrenal/thyroid health)
- Immune system support
- Antioxidant, anti-inflammatory, anti-cancer, and anti-tumor

Opinions vary as to whether chrysin has an effect on estrogen levels. It is possible that the benefits derived from the consumption of chrysin are due to it being a flavonoid. Flavonoids possess antioxidant and anti-inflammatory properties.

The nutritional supplement chrysin is promoted as an aromatase inhibitor. It should be noted that aromatase inhibitors (and estrogen blockers) have no effect on xenoestrogens. We ingest xenoestrogenic substances on a daily basis and these must be flushed out on a daily basis which is why detoxifying foods, herbs and nutritional supplements are ideal for the job.

NOTE

Do not consume with sugar or sweeteners. Sugar and sweeteners are counter effective to hormonal balance.

LEARN MORE

Chrysin - Wikipedia, the free encyclopedia
http://en.wikipedia.org/wiki/Chrysin
Passiflora - Wikipedia, the free encyclopedia
http://en.wikipedia.org/wiki/Passion_flower
Passiflora edulis - Wikipedia, the free encyclopedia
http://en.wikipedia.org/wiki/Passion_fruit
Passion fruit | Phytochemicals
http://www.phytochemicals.info/plants/passion-fruit.php

T NATION | Naturally Occurring Aromatase Inhibitors
http://www.t-nation.com/readArticle.do?id=460290&cr=supplements%E2%80%8E

Chrysin: Is It An Effective Aromatase Inhibitor? | Ward Dean, MD
http://warddeanmd.com/chrysin-is-it-an-effective-aromatase-inhibitor/

Chrysin – Research – LifeOne
http://www.lifeone.org/chrysin.html

Aromatase Inhibitors – are there natural alternatives to the breast cancer drugs? | Cancer Active
http://www.canceractive.com/cancer-active-page-link.aspx?n=2412

Natural Aromatase Inhibitor herbal supplements - Ray Sahelian, M.D.
www.raysahelian.com/aromatase.html

Piperine - Wikipedia, the free encyclopedia
http://en.wikipedia.org/wiki/Piperine

The 14 Most Valuable Cures from the Miracle Doctor
https://images.web-purchases.com/Library-1500034/600RNAHPDF_NAHUpsellPremiums.pdf

Flavonoid inhibition of aromatase enzyme activity in human preadipocytes | Science Direct
http://www.sciencedirect.com/science/article/pii/0960076093902280

Chrysin Review: Does Chrysin Work As An Estrogen Blocker? | Ultimate Fat Burner
http://bodybuilding.ultimatefatburner.com/chrysin-review.html

Chrysin supplement benefit | Chrysin.mobi
http://www.chrysin.mobi/

Chrysin is Natural Alternative to Toxic Breast Cancer Drugs | Natural News
http://www.naturalnews.com/026086_cancer_drug_chrysin.html#

Effects of chrysin on urinary testosterone levels in human males. | ncbi.nlm.nih.gov
http://www.ncbi.nlm.nih.gov/pubmed/14977449

Facile synthesis of chrysin-derivatives with promising activities as aromatase inhibitors. | ncbi.nlm.nih.gov
http://www.ncbi.nlm.nih.gov/pubmed/21366040

Sexual Functioning in Men can be Fully Restored Naturally | Natural News
http://www.naturalnews.com/026219_testosterone_rats_body.html

Bodybuilding.com - Clayton's Health Facts: Chrysin.
http://www.bodybuilding.com/fun/southfacts_chrysin.htm

Hefty dose of chrysin boosts testosterone synthesis | Ergo Log
http://www.ergo-log.com/chrysin-boosts-testosterone-synthesis.html

LE Magazine, January 2000 - Cover Story: Replenish Testosterone Naturally — Plant extracts favorably alter hormone metabolism and improve sexual desire in men
http://www.lef.org/magazine/mag2000/jan00-cover2.htm

With a healthy gut, one would effectively absorb all the necessary nutrients needed for detoxification through one's diet. Eating healthy organic food in a mindful, relaxed way may be one of the more critical steps along with supporting the GI tract for metabolizing xenoestrogens.

What are xenoestrogens and their impact on your health? | Flowing Health
http://flowinghealth.org/xenoestrogen_patient_handout.pdf

CITRULLINE

Although the chemicals in our cosmetics do constitute a low risk in the sense that they won't cause any immediate damage, continuous accumulation of these low doses can cause reproductive problems. For instance, phthalates and PCBs were found to cause infertility in both men and women, early puberty in girls, and early menopause in women. There's a high chance that your early perimenopause symptoms are caused by the cosmetics you use.

Perimenopause - Natural Cosmetics Are a Must | Ezine Articles

http://ezinearticles.com/?Perimenopause---Natural-Cosmetics-Are-a-Must&id=4569736

Citrulline is an amino acid (protein). Related amino acids are arginine and ornithine. All three can be found in various sports and libido enhancement supplements. The consumption of these amino acids is said to improve circulation and the engorgement capacity of erectile tissues.

CITRULLINE USES

- Sexual and reproductive function
- Gastrointestinal health
- Rest and recovery support, athletic and otherwise
- Vitality, energy, and stamina
- Cardiovascular health
- Detoxification
- Weight management

The best known food source of citrulline is watermelon rind. Watermelon rind can be sliced or chopped and added to salads, pressed into a juice, or blended as a part of a smoothie.

Other sources of citrulline include the rest of the melon family, cucumber, onion family, and protein-rich foods (meat, fish, poultry, beans, nuts, etc.).

NOTE

Do not consume with sugar or sweeteners. Sugar and sweeteners are counter effective to hormonal balance.

NOTE 2

When eating the skins and rinds of fruits and veggies make sure that these are all organic, non-GMO, and grown in mineral-rich, organic soils.

LEARN MORE

Oral L-citrulline supplementation improves erection hardness in men with mild erectile dysfunction. [Urology. 2011] - PubMed - NCBI
http://www.ncbi.nlm.nih.gov/pubmed/21195829
Citrulline - Wikipedia, the free encyclopedia
http://en.wikipedia.org/wiki/Citrulline
Benefits of Watermelon Rinds | LIVESTRONG.COM
http://www.livestrong.com/article/408893-benefits-of-watermelon-rinds/

6 Hidden Health Benefits of Eating Peels, Stems and Rinds | Oprah
http://www.oprah.com/health/Nutritional-Benefits-of-Eating-Peels-Stems-and-Rinds

Nature's Viagra - Watermelon Rind Juice :-) - YouTube
http://youtu.be/TADnG60QYwM

Bodybuilding.com - Give L-Citrulline Some Consideration For Greater Performance In The Gym!
http://www.bodybuilding.com/fun/l_citrulline_increases_performance.htm

The Best Time to Take L-Citrulline | LIVESTRONG.COM
http://www.livestrong.com/article/553630-the-best-time-to-take-l-citrulline/

L-Citrulline and L-Arginine: This One-Two Amino Acid Punch Can Improve Circulation And Your Love Life | Smart Publications
http://www.smart-publications.com/articles/l-citrulline-and-l-arginine-this-one-two-amino-acid-punch-can-improve-

Citrulline Benefits | Peak Testosterone
http://www.peaktestosterone.com/Citrulline_Benefits.aspx

L-Citrulline's Many Benefits | Anti Aging Prime
http://www.antiagingprime.com/l-citrullinesman.html

Erectile Dysfunction – Supplements | Peak Testosterone
http://www.peaktestosterone.com/Erectile_Supplements.aspx

Sexy Supplements | Muscle & Performance Magazine
http://www.muscleandperformancemag.com/nutrition-supplements/2011/11/sexy-supplements

Why you should take citrulline | Pill Scout
http://www.pillscout.com/2013/05/20/why-you-should-take-citrulline/

142

Citrulline malate enhances athletic anaerobic performance and relieves muscle soreness. [J Strength Cond Res. 2010] - PubMed - NCBI
http://www.ncbi.nlm.nih.gov/pubmed/20386132
My Citrulline Malate Experiment | Muscle Evo
http://muscleevo.net/citrulline-malate/#.U5PkkXJdWSo
A Libido Boosting Sex Smoothie For Your Sexual Health | Man of Vigor
http://www.manofvigor.com/body/libido-boosting-sex-smoothie-sexual-health/
Foods Containing L-Citrulline | LIVESTRONG.COM
http://www.livestrong.com/article/321823-foods-containing-citrulline/

Hormones are also not being prescribed properly. For example, some women use prescriptions of a combination of estrogen, progesterone and testosterone all together in a cream applied every day when these hormones should be applied separately. Testosterone, for instance, should be applied just above the clitoris where hair grows and this is because testosterone creams can cause hair growth if applied repeatedly to the same location. Testosterone is generally applied every day for seven days, then once or twice a week thereafter.
Hormone Help Issue 34 | Healthy Immunity
http://www.healthyimmunity.com/newsletter/034.asp

The Natural Path to Hormonal Wellness, Part 1 by Katarina Nolte
Pages: 201 (23,609 words); Copyright © 2014 by Katarina Nolte.
All rights reserved. http://katarinanolte.com/ July 2014

D-ASPARTIC ACID

Anytime one increases testosterone there is the follow on effect of raising estrogen. This happens whether you inject exogenous test, HcG, take Clomid or Tamoxifin, take Alpha Male (for those who respond to this)....anything that raises your hormone levels. ... In this case, increased T always results in increased E depending on YOUR body's physiological make up (if you have higher aromatase than another, of course you're going to have more T to E conversion).

TESTOSTERONE NATION | D-Aspartic Acid - Page 1
http://tnation.t-nation.com/free_online_forum/sports_body_training_performance_bodybuilding_thibaudeau/daspartic_acid_

D-aspartic acid is an amino acid (protein). D-aspartic acid is said to raise LH (luteinizing hormone) which is associated with higher free (bioavailable) testosterone levels. Paradoxically, d-aspartic acid is also believed to cause an increase in aromatase levels.

D-ASPARTIC ACID USES

- Sexual and reproductive function
- Rest and recovery support, athletic and otherwise

Aspartic acid is found in protein-rich foods (meat, fish, poultry, beans, nuts, etc.), sprouts, avocado, asparagus, and seaweeds.

Note

Do not consume with sugar or sweeteners. Sugar and sweeteners are counter effective to hormonal balance.

Note 2

When consumed in combination, amino acids tend to compete with one another for absorption, which is why individual amino acids are sold in powder, liquid, capsule and tablet form at health food stores as well as online.

LEARN MORE

Three grams D-aspartic acid raises testosterone levels by forty percent | Ergo Log
http://www.ergo-log.com/dasparticacidtestosterone.html
TESTOSTERONE NATION | D-Aspartic Acid - Page 1
http://tnation.t-nation.com/free_online_forum/sports_body_training_pe rformance_bodybuilding_thibaudeau/daspartic_acid_
Aspartic acid - Wikipedia, the free encyclopedia
http://en.wikipedia.org/wiki/Aspartic_acid
Foods High in D-Aspartic Acid | LIVESTRONG.COM
http://www.livestrong.com/article/518754-foods-high-in-d-aspartic-acid/
When Hype Meets Reality: D-Aspartic Acid Turns Out to Be Another Supplemental Nonstarter in First Human Trial With Any Relevance for Healthy Young Men - SuppVersity
http://suppversity.blogspot.com/2013/08/when-hype-meets-reality-d-aspartic-acid.html

D-aspartic acid supplementation combined with 28 days of heavy resistance training has no effect on body composition, muscle strength, and serum hormones associated with the hypothalamo-pituitary-gonadal axis in resistance-trained men. - PubMed - NCBI

http://www.ncbi.nlm.nih.gov/pubmed/24074738

The more raw food that the women eat, the more likely they are to have partial or total amenorrhea. Males eating a raw diet might also notice a change in reproductive hormones, primarily a decrease in testosterone production.
Precision Nutrition » All About Raw Food
http://www.precisionnutrition.com/all-about-raw-food

The Natural Path to Hormonal Wellness, Part 1 by Katarina Nolte
Pages: 201 (23,609 words); Copyright © 2014 by Katarina Nolte.
All rights reserved. http://katarinanolte.com/ July 2014

AUTHOR

"The Natural Path to Hormonal Wellness, Part 1"
is my fourth book on the subject of wellness after
"So Long Constipation, Part 1", "100 Steps to a
Lean Body", and "49 Gluten-free Recipes".

Next, I will be concluding the Gluten-free Recipe
Book Series, followed by "So Long Constipation,
Part 2".

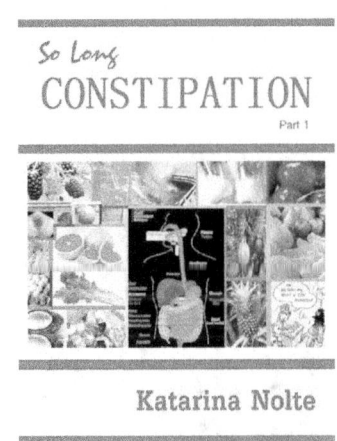

The Natural Path to Hormonal Wellness, Part 1 by Katarina Nolte
Pages: 201 (23,609 words); Copyright © 2014 by Katarina Nolte.
All rights reserved. http://katarinanolte.com/ July 2014

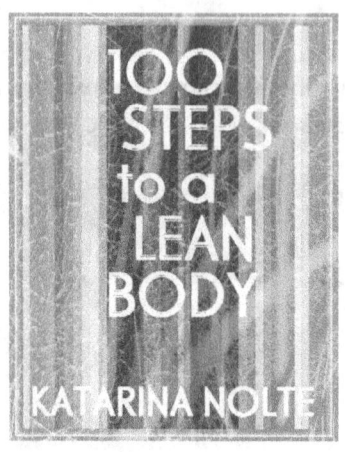

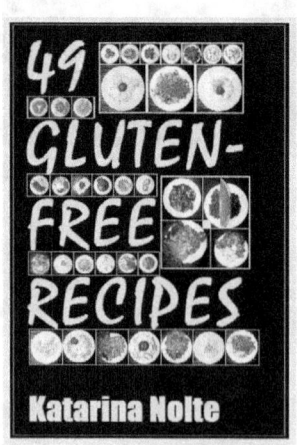

The Natural Path to Hormonal Wellness, Part 1 by Katarina Nolte
Pages: 201 (23,609 words); Copyright © 2014 by Katarina Nolte.
All rights reserved. http://katarinanolte.com/ July 2014

AFTERTHOUGHT

I hope you found **"The Natural Path to Hormonal Wellness, Part 1"** to be a practical and informative read and would appreciate it if you could take a moment to post a review.

Website: http://katarinanolte.com/

Mobile: http://m.katarinanolte.com/

Blog: http://katarinanolte.com/WordPressBlog/

Newsletter: http://katarinanolte.com/WordPressBlog/MailChimp

Follow me on Twitter @KatarinaNolte and connect with me on LinkedIn (http://www.linkedin.com/in/katarinanolte).

The Natural Path to Hormonal Wellness, Part 1 by Katarina Nolte
Pages: 201 (23,609 words); Copyright © 2014 by Katarina Nolte.
All rights reserved. http://katarinanolte.com/ July 2014

RECOMMENDED RESOURCES

Prescription for Herbal Healing, 2nd Edition: An Easy-to-Use A-to-Z Reference to Hundreds of Common Disorders and Their Herbal Remedies | Phyllis A. Balch CNC, Stacey Bell
http://www.amazon.com/Prescription-Herbal-Healing-Easy---Use/dp/1583334521/

PDR for Herbal Medicines, 4th Edition | Thomson Healthcare
http://www.amazon.com/PDR-Herbal-Medicines-4th-Edition/dp/1563636786

Bulk Organic Herbs & Spices – Mountain Rose Herbs
https://www.mountainroseherbs.com/catalog/herbs/bulk

Raintree Nutrition Herbal Supplements and Formulas
http://www.rain-tree.com/rtmprod.htm#.U7PbDZRdWSo

Herbs A-Z: Find the widest selection of high-quality culinary, wellness and craft herbs available. | Frontier Coop
http://www.frontiercoop.com/prodlist.php?ct=hchhaz

The Natural Path to Hormonal Wellness, Part 1 by Katarina Nolte
Pages: 201 (23,609 words); Copyright © 2014 by Katarina Nolte.
All rights reserved. http://katarinanolte.com/ July 2014

ADDITIONAL RESOURCES

Hormonal Imbalance & the Modern Lifestyle | Macabido
http://macabido.com/modern-lifestyles-hormonal-imbalance/

GMO Corn & Roundup Shown to Cause Hormonal Imbalance | Natural Fertility Info
http://natural-fertility-info.com/gmo-corn-hormonal-imbalance.html

146 Reasons Why Sugar Is Ruining Your Health | Rheumatic
http://rheumatic.org/sugar.htm

Hormonal Imbalance Caused by Alcoholism | Alcohol Rehab
http://alcoholrehab.com/alcoholism/hormonal-imbalance-caused-by-alcoholism/

The Candida Link: Hormonal Imbalance and the Natural Way To Remedy PMS and Improve Your Health | Candida Hormonal Imbalance | Body Ecology
http://candidahormonalimbalance.bodyecology.com/

The Hidden Causes Behind Hormonal Imbalances | VRP
http://www.vrp.com/hormone-support/the-hidden-causes-behind-hormonal-imbalances

Hormonal Influences on the Gastrointestinal Tract and Irritable Bowel Syndrome | Weill Cornell Physicians
http://weillcornell.org/pdf/ibs/Frissora_-_Practical_GastroHORMONES.pdf

The Natural Path to Hormonal Wellness, Part 1 by Katarina Nolte
Pages: 201 (23,609 words); Copyright © 2014 by Katarina Nolte.
All rights reserved. http://katarinanolte.com/ July 2014

Gut and hormones and obesity. [Front Horm Res. 2008] - PubMed - NCBI
http://www.ncbi.nlm.nih.gov/pubmed/18230902

Hormone imbalances hindering your weight-loss efforts - Chatelaine
http://www.chatelaine.com/health/wellness/imbalances-halting-your-weight-loss/

Obesity Linked To Hormone Imbalance That Impacts Sexual Quality Of Life – Science Daily
http://www.sciencedaily.com/releases/2009/03/090303082815.htm

Weight gain and hormone imbalances - they always go hand in hand! │ Susan Riegg MD
http://www.susanrieggmd.com/weight-gain/

The Impact of Obesity On Thyroid Health │ Natural Endocrine Solutions
http://www.naturalendocrinesolutions.com/articles/the-impact-of-obesity-on-thyroid-health/

HowStuffWorks "Hormone Imbalances and Infertility"
http://health.howstuffworks.com/pregnancy-and-parenting/pregnancy/fertility/hormone-imbalances-and-infertility1.htm

Infertility Rates on the Rise - Hormonal Imbalances - India - YouTube
http://youtu.be/gIoC-H2QWrg

Causes of Male Infertility: What You Need to Know │ Natural Fertility Info
http://natural-fertility-info.com/causes-of-male-infertility-what-you-need-to-know.html

Oxidative stress and male infertility—a clinical perspective │ Human Reproductive Update │ Oxford Journals
http://humupd.oxfordjournals.org/content/14/3/243.full

152

Pollutants Linked to Lower Fertility in Both Men and Women | TIME.com

http://healthland.time.com/2012/11/15/pollutants-linked-to-lower-fertility-in-both-men-and-women/

Declining Male Fertility Linked To Water Pollution – Science Daily

http://www.sciencedaily.com/releases/2009/01/090118200636.htm

Male fertility decline in China linked to air pollution | Luna Lin - China Dialogue

https://www.chinadialogue.net/blog/6523-Male-fertility-decline-in-China-linked-to-air-pollution/en

Testosterone levels have fallen in American men over the past 2 decades

http://www.ourstolenfuture.org/newscience/reproduction/2006/2006-1210travisonetal.html

Evidence for decreasing quality of semen during past 50 years. | ncbi.nlm.nih.gov

http://www.ncbi.nlm.nih.gov/pmc/articles/PMC1883354/

The UltraMind Solution: Key #2 Balance Your Hormones - Dr. Mark Hyman

http://drhyman.com/blog/2012/01/27/the-ultramind-solution-key-2-balance-your-hormones/#close

Female hormone imbalance could be to blame for male obesity in Western nations: study | Health & Wellbeing | Nine MSN

http://health.ninemsn.com.au/article.aspx?id=8861187

Sex effects of water pollution - Wikipedia, the free encyclopedia

http://en.wikipedia.org/wiki/Sex_effects_of_water_pollution

Common Signs of Hormone Imbalances - Euphoric Roots

http://euphoricroots.com/common-signs-of-hormone-imbalances/

The Natural Path to Hormonal Wellness, Part 1 by Katarina Nolte
Pages: 201 (23,609 words); Copyright © 2014 by Katarina Nolte.
All rights reserved. http://katarinanolte.com/ July 2014

Surprise bonus gift...

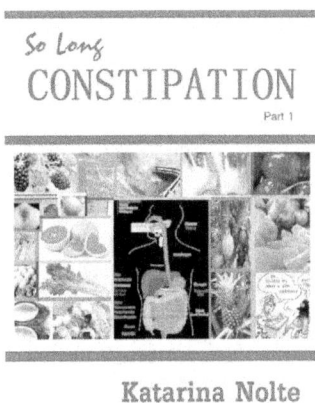

So Long
CONSTIPATION
Part 1

Katarina Nolte

Chapter One: Constipation

Most people think that they are not constipated if they are having one bowel movement a day. Yet, we eat three meals a day. Where are the other two meals going if they're not being eliminated through the colon? The answer actually is somewhat frightening. The rest of the food that is not absorbed by the body as nutrients stays around the body in unlikely places -- against the colon walls, in tissues and organs, in arteries -- any place at all in the body can serve as a receptacle for uneliminated waste.

Keeping your colon clean | Natural News
http://www.naturalnews.com/033165_colon_cleansing_health.html

The Natural Path to Hormonal Wellness, Part 1 by Katarina Nolte
Pages: 201 (23,609 words); Copyright © 2014 by Katarina Nolte.
All rights reserved. http://katarinanolte.com/ July 2014

Cognizance

First, an estimated 90 percent of the population has a problem with candida overgrowth, although most don't know it.
Antibiotics Cause Cancer? | Huffingtong Post
http://www.huffingtonpost.com/kim-evans/antibiotics-cause-cancer_b_186968.html

So Long Constipation, Part 1 is about much more than constipation. The reason is very simple: once you get rid of constipation you will not only want to remain constipation-free, but also continue to increase your newly regained wellbeing. This will take time and the willingness to learn more on the subject.

To be consistently successful on this road, it is best to try one thing at a time, and see how well it can be integrated into your lifestyle and schedule, as well as how it suits your individually unique mind-body chemistry.

Regardless of the degree or frequency of the constipation and related ailments, it is important not to skip any parts of So Long Constipation, Part 1 that may not appear to apply and instead read this book in its entirety.

Our bodies are not manmade engines which can be taken apart and repaired or replaced part by part. The human body, or the body of any mammal for that matter, is a complex system in which internal and external actions must work in concert in order for us to function and feel our best, regardless of age and other factors. What we consume and how we consume it, along with our general awareness

The Natural Path to Hormonal Wellness, Part 1 by Katarina Nolte
Pages: 201 (23,609 words); Copyright © 2014 by Katarina Nolte.
All rights reserved. http://katarinanolte.com/ July 2014

and attitude, are the most essential components of this process.

The more clearly we see the connection between consumption and function (or dysfunction), food and wellbeing, the more competent we become at replacing discomfort with wellness.

When it comes to constipation, one thing can lead to another, and before we know it, we realize that we are no longer enjoying optimal health. The constipation chain reaction can begin with the commonly known symptoms such as incomplete evacuation, straining, pain, discomfort, stools not passing easily, hard stools, dry stools, tiny stools, infrequent bowel movements, urge to go and then nothing, etc. This obvious failure to eliminate thoroughly can then lead to things like gas, cellulite, hernia, hemorrhoids, varicose veins, indigestion, weight gain, diverticulitis, insomnia, headaches, cancer, compacted fecal matter, bad breath, body odor, depression, fatigue, pain, abdominal cramps, bloating, weight gain, headaches, backaches, appendicitis, polyposis, neuropathy, megacolon, irritable bowel (IBS), inflammatory bowel disease (IBD), premenstrual syndrome (PMS), menstrual cramps, appendicitis, ulcers, chronic inflammation, internal bleeding, anal fissures, etc. And it all begins due to the lack of knowledge, like what to eat and what to avoid, and that, ideally, one should have between one and five easy and smooth bowel movements every single day.

Did You Poop Today? | Global Healing Center
http://www.globalhealingcenter.com/constipation-and-colon-cleansing/poop

Constipation | Wikipedia
http://en.wikipedia.org/wiki/Constipation
**Constipation | National Digestive Diseases
Information Clearinghouse (NDDIC)**
http://digestive.niddk.nih.gov/ddiseases/pubs/constipation/
**If you suffer from chronic or periodic constipation
we have some pointers on how to have natural
healthy regular bowel movements. | Ageless.co.za**
http://www.ageless.co.za/constipation.htm#Stress

*Constipation rarely happens out of the blue in
otherwise healthy adults. It is usually preceded by
decades of semi-regular stools that are either too
large, or too hard, or both. These abnormal stools
cause gradual nerve damage and enlargement of
the colon, rectum, and hemorrhoidal pads until one
day the bowels refuse to move as was meant by
nature — once or twice daily, usually after a meal,
and with zero effort or notice.*
**Frequently Asked Questions: Constipation | Gut
Sense**
http://www.gutsense.org/constipation/faq.html

The Natural Path to Hormonal Wellness, Part 1 by Katarina Nolte
Pages: 201 (23,609 words); Copyright © 2014 by Katarina Nolte.
All rights reserved. http://katarinanolte.com/ July 2014

Cradle to Grave

*New research shows that soy oil makes for an
amazing lubricant for skateboards or door hinges,
while soybeans provide a fantastic insect repellent.
Mosquitoes avoid it like the plague.*
**The selling of Frankensoy© What Doctors Don't Tell
You | Healthy.net**
http://www.healthy.net/scr/article.aspx?Id=7746

Due to our typically unnatural diet and lifestyle,
constipation is a slowly evolving dysfunction of the
gastrointestinal system beginning in infancy and
progressing as we age and is accompanied by other
symptoms of digestive deterioration.

The path from constipation to neurological
degeneration includes malnutrition (nutrient-poor
diet), malabsorption of nutrients, and toxin
reabsorption (from stool). This is particularly
devastating for infants and children whose growth
and development depend on the amounts of
nutrients they receive. Similarly, the aging
population (40+) requires complete and proper
digestion as their slowing systems struggle to
maintain homeostasis.

One of the most important steps that must be
taken in order to eliminate constipation for good is
to revive our taste buds, which just like our
olfactory (sense of smell) become desensitized when
bombarded by artificial substances. While our
sense of smell is weakened by industrial perfumes,
deodorants, deodorizers, etc., our taste buds (and
our olfactory system) suffer due to exposure to
pesticides, fungicides, herbicides, additives (incl.

flavors), colors and dyes, leading to the inability to fully taste and enjoy natural foods. The compromised taste and smell functions distort our instinctive ability to crave and choose foods our bodies need for optimal function.

Further, our primal instincts are tricked by a new, 5th 'taste' (fresh from the laboratory), called 'umami' or 'savory'. It is the taste of none other than monosodium glutamate (MSG), commonly found in restaurant food, frozen meals, dried meals, canned foods, and other ready to eat preparations.

Aside from a truly natural diet, cleansing, once again, is critical for the regeneration of the senses as these require optimal function of our various glands (along with the rest of the internal system).

Digestive System | Jon Barron
http://www.jonbarron.org/enzymes/digestive-health-acid-reflux-ulcers
Olfactory system | Wikipedia
http://en.wikipedia.org/wiki/Olfactory_system
Umami | Wikipedia
http://en.wikipedia.org/wiki/Umami
Frequently Asked Questions: Constipation | Gut Sense
http://www.gutsense.org/constipation/faq.html
What Is The Connection Between Infant Constipation, Diarrhea, and Autism? | Gut Sense
http://www.gutsense.org/constipation/autism.html
Do Artificial Flavors Spoil Us For the Taste of Real Food? | NY Times
http://www.nytimes.com/1996/01/03/garden/do-artificial-flavors-spoil-us-for-the-taste-of-real-food.html
Flavor | Wikipedia
https://en.wikipedia.org/wiki/Flavor

Up to 75% of what we perceive as taste is due to smell.

Digestive System | Jon Barron

http://www.jonbarron.org/enzymes/digestive-health-acid-reflux-ulcers

Canal

It is really true that the mouth of a dog that drinks from the toilet is cleaner than yours. And if you must be bitten, better to be bitten by a dog than a person.
Digestive System | Jon Barron
http://www.jonbarron.org/enzymes/digestive-health-acid-reflux-ulcers

Digestion begins in the nose, which alerts us to the presence of food and tells us what to eat. It continues in the mouth, where it is assisted by taste buds and enzyme-rich saliva. Expert opinion varies when it comes to the question of whether the human jaw is that of an omnivore (eats everything), a frugivore (mostly fruitarian), or a carnivore (mega meat lover).

From the mouth, food passes through the esophagus, and lands in the stomach. Digestion is assisted by the liver, kidneys, the gallbladder, the bile duct, and the pancreas.

Finally in the small intestine, nutrient absorption takes place with the help of beneficial gut bacteria and digestive enzymes. The rest of the content is indigestible stuff and includes metabolic waste, pharmaceuticals, heavy metals, and the various inedible factory food additives. In addition, it is in the gut where stuff we absorb from water, air, and cosmetics, is processed and eliminated, which, in turn, makes digestive (gut cleansing) and extra-digestive (sweating, exercise, meditation) cleansing so crucial, along with a natural diet/lifestyle.

A healthy pancreas is crucial for optimal digestive functioning, because it is the pancreas that

The Natural Path to Hormonal Wellness, Part 1 by Katarina Nolte
Pages: 201 (23,609 words); Copyright © 2014 by Katarina Nolte.
All rights reserved. http://katarinanolte.com/ July 2014

regulates blood sugar, and produces enzymes essential for proper digestion of food and the absorption of vital nutrients. Industrially processed food overworks the pancreas, so that, over time, digestive and extradigestive health issues arise. These are: tummy ache, nausea, malabsorption, constipation, low energy, itchy skin, jaundice, cellular starvation, as well as diabetes and related cardiovascular and neurological problems.

Is It Your Stomach or Is It Your Pancreas That's Causing Pain? | Natural News
http://www.NaturalNews.com/023161_pancreas_health_insulin.html
Digestive System | Jon Barron
http://www.jonbarron.org/enzymes/digestive-health-acid-reflux-ulcers
Human as Frugivore | Whale.to
http://www.whale.to/a/frugivore_h.html
The Fruitarian Worldwide Network
http://www.fruitnet.org/

Sometimes after any type of abdominal surgery scar tissue will grow internally and pinch off or restrict a section of your bowel.
Did You Poop Today? | Global Healing Center
http://www.globalhealingcenter.com/constipation-and-colon-cleansing/poop

The Natural Path to Hormonal Wellness, Part 1 by Katarina Nolte
Pages: 201 (23,609 words); Copyright © 2014 by Katarina Nolte.
All rights reserved. http://katarinanolte.com/ July 2014

Missing

The Chinese did not eat unfermented soybean products.

THE PLOY OF SOY - Enzyme Inhibitors | Consumer Health

http://www.consumerhealth.org/articles/display.cfm?ID=20000501001338

Chronic constipation often leads to high blood pressure and heart problems. Women are more likely to suffer from constipation and cardiovascular problems due to industrial toxins (air, water, food, and manmade products), anatomy (uterus), pregnancy, iatrogenic illness, chronic stress, lack of exercise, malabsorption, and nutritional deficiencies (enzymes, friendly gut bacteria, antioxidants, protein, magnesium, trace elements, and healthy oils).

Constipation can be caused by unforeseen events affecting the mind (unexpected event) or the entire mind-body system (travel, accident, etc.) in a stressful manner.

It can also be caused by industrially processed food, food allergies and intolerances, a sedentary lifestyle and consequential muscular weakness, pharmaceuticals, alcohol, anal sex, dry climate, and advanced age (70+).

Constipation can as well be a symptom of a given disease or a side effect of the treatment of a disease (surgery, anesthetics and other meds, colonoscopy, scar tissue, missing organs, radiation, etc.).

A less known type of constipation is caused by improper prioritization. Rather than going to the

The Natural Path to Hormonal Wellness, Part 1 by Katarina Nolte
Pages: 201 (23,609 words); Copyright © 2014 by Katarina Nolte.
All rights reserved. http://katarinanolte.com/ July 2014

bathroom when we feel the urge, we postpone the deed, thereby training the body to discontinue bowel movement signaling. And then, when we finally go to the bathroom, nothing happens, causing the stool to linger and dry up, and making it difficult to expel the next time we do go to the bathroom when nature calls. Long term, this can cause chronic or even acute constipation.

People can also be constipated for no apparent reason. A general attitude that is on the restricted, restrained side due to unresolved issues, can translate into repressed bodily functioning.

Different Types of Constipation | Articles Base
http://www.articlesbase.com/alternative-medicine-articles/different-types-of-constipation-588948.html
Stress may take two paths in depression - endogenous and reactive depression | Find Articles
http://findarticles.com/p/articles/mi_m1200/is_n4_v146/ai_15657596/
Is Constipation Stressing Your Heart Out? | Recipe to Health
http://recipetohealth.com/uncategorized/is-constipation-stressing-your-heart-out-here%e2%80%99s-6-ways-to-avoid-constipation/
Iatrogenic – Definition | The Free Dictionary
http://www.thefreedictionary.com/iatrogenic
Death by Medicine–Iatrogenic illness | Sustainable Medicine
http://sustainablemedicine.org/2008/10/death-by-medicine-iatrogenic-illness/

The Natural Path to Hormonal Wellness, Part 1 by Katarina Nolte
Pages: 201 (23,609 words); Copyright © 2014 by Katarina Nolte.
All rights reserved. http://katarinanolte.com/ July 2014

Recognition of the psychosomatic factors that influence the etiology of constipation. Finally, psychology plays a huge role in constipation because the very last act of moving the bowels — letting it go — can be controlled and... suppressed at will. Sure, the ability to withhold moving the bowels is an absolutely essential trait for city dwellers, but, unfortunately, taken too far, it is behind many cases of chronic constipation.

Frequently Asked Questions: Constipation | Gut Sense

http://www.gutsense.org/constipation/faq.html

The Natural Path to Hormonal Wellness, Part 1 by Katarina Nolte
Pages: 201 (23,609 words); Copyright © 2014 by Katarina Nolte.
All rights reserved. http://katarinanolte.com/ July 2014

Spine

Constipation occurs when the waste material becomes blocked in the lower intestine. The blockage can cause pressure in the lower back. The pain will get worse if the impaction isn't eliminated. That's because your body continues to produce waste material even if it's not passing it. Conversely, back pain from lifting, a sudden jerk, or other straining activities can cause a bout of constipation. That's due to the fact that the muscles in the lower back in spasm can interfere with the autonomic nerves responsible for peristalsis of bowel movements.

Constipation and Back Pain | Global Healing Center
http://www.globalhealingcenter.com/back-pain-constipation.html

Constipation can cause back pain and vice versa. Both health issues are most common among women and people over the age of 30. Constipation is however not the sole culprit causing back pain, but rather the fact that constipated individuals' systems carry a backlog of metabolic wastes of all sorts. Most toxins have a neurotoxic effect raking havoc on the spinal part of the central nervous system, among other things. Additionally, a stuffed colon may be causing pressure, which results in back pain and discomfort. Excessive straining during difficult bowel movements can further exacerbate the situation, as can weak or unbalanced muscles (back, buttocks, waist, hip, and abdominal muscles).

The Natural Path to Hormonal Wellness, Part 1 by Katarina Nolte
Pages: 201 (23,609 words); Copyright © 2014 by Katarina Nolte.
All rights reserved. http://katarinanolte.com/ July 2014

Back pain constipation is often related to mental-,
spiritual-, or emotional stress which can be
gradually alleviated with regular practice of
relaxing activities like meditation, stretching,
music therapy, dancing, aromatherapy, light
therapy (preferably outdoors), walking and/or semi
jogging (walk-jog-walk), and various types of
nature therapy like gardening or hiking.
Furthermore, slow tempo exercise leads to more
intense deep tissue (muscle directly attached to
bone) strengthening with less pressure on the
joints/spine and an increased emphasis on
posture and execution.

**Back Pain Constipation | Colon Cleanse
Constipation**
http://www.colon-cleanse-constipation.com/back-
pain-constipation.html
**Why Nature Is Therapeutic | Wilderness Program
Info**
http://www.wilderness-programs-info.com/nature-is-
therapeutic.html
Fast vs Slow: Tempo demystified | The Swole
http://theswole.com/general/fast-vs-slow/
Muscle weakness | Wikipedia
http://en.wikipedia.org/wiki/Muscle_weakness
Spiritual Stress - Stress Management | Net Places
http://www.netplaces.com/stress-management/what-
is-stress-doing-to-me/stress-on-your-spirit.htm

The Natural Path to Hormonal Wellness, Part 1 by Katarina Nolte
Pages: 201 (23,609 words); Copyright © 2014 by Katarina Nolte.
All rights reserved. http://katarinanolte.com/ July 2014

Fiber is ok to digest as long as food does not contain too much of it. Unlike pigeons, we do not have a crop in which we can pre-digest cereals. And unlike cows, we do not have 4 stomachs to gradually ferment vegetables and grasses. Our bowels do not like excessive fiber. 'Foods' containing much fiber make your bowels age much faster.
Food Causing Constipation │ 13 Waisays
http://www.13.waisays.com/constipation.htm

Roughage

*Environmental toxins modify our genes and affect
our children and grandchildren; enormous
implications for risk assessment of synthetic
chemical and other xenobiotics.*
Epigenetic Toxicology | I-SIS.org.uk
http://www.i-sis.org.uk/epigeneticToxicology.php

The most important thing to know about fiber in
relation to constipation is that fiber is found in
plant foods, and that it is the plant foods that are
healthy for digestion, not the fiber per se. This is
because plant foods contain many other health
supporting nutrients, which together with soluble
(digestible) fiber stimulate proper digestion. The
popular idea of roughage solving the problem of
constipation is entirely incorrect, as roughage
tends to do the very opposite.

Many plant foods consist of both, soluble
(digestible) and insoluble (indigestible) fiber, and
should therefore be avoided until constipation has
been eliminated. Plants with indigestible fiber are
primarily those which require soaking and/or
cooking prior to consumption, like grains, beans,
corn, nuts, and seeds.

Indigestible parts of plant foods can damage the
digestive function and microbial balance, leading to
bloating, gas, indigestion, constipation, etc.

Further, excessive consumption of starchy
carbohydrates (grains, corn, beans, and rice) leads
to excess fiber and blood sugar, which then lead to
digestive-, weight-, and skin problems (as a
starter).

170

The Natural Path to Hormonal Wellness, Part 1 by Katarina Nolte
Pages: 201 (23,609 words); Copyright © 2014 by Katarina Nolte.
All rights reserved. http://katarinanolte.com/ July 2014

And finally, one of the main reasons why roughage is a really bad idea when one is constipated is that it bulks up the stool which had a hard time passing to begin with. Cramps, discomfort, and exhaustion follow, due to the fact that fat absorption is compromised. Essential fat-soluble vitamins and minerals now cannot be utilized by the body. This malabsorption and malnutrition then lead to immunity-, endocrine-, cardiovascular-, connective tissue-, and weight problems.

People who suffer from constipation are often unable to digest many vegetables. In such cases, a balanced consumption of salad vegetables, cooked cruciferous veggies, and most of all freshly pressed fruit or vegetable juices, solves the problem.

Once again, the benefits of fiber are limited to soluble (digestible) fiber in combination with the countless nutrients found primarily in fresh, preferably organic, or at least local, fruits and vegetables.

Constipation is often either caused by, related to, or the cause of inflammation, which in turn aggravates some or all vital systems and functions. Fruits and vegetables, as well as freshly pressed juices thereof clear up the system, beat inflammation, and strengthen immunity, especially when consumed together with healthy fats (olive, coconut, fish, grape, and flax).

One of the consequences of eating inedible 'foods' like insoluble fiber, factory food (most of which is grain-, corn-, and/or soy-based), and laboratory spices (additives, preservatives, dyes, etc.), is the loss of healthy gut microbes, an overgrowth of unhealthy gut microbes, and an accumulation of metabolic wastes (undigested food, microbial waste products, etc.). Such a state, in turn, leads to an increase in inflammation and all types of ills and ails in the gut and beyond. The chaotically functioning gut will produce constipation, diarrhea, fungal infections, and autoimmune diseases.

An Apple a Day? Study Shows Soluble Fiber Boosts Immune System │ Science Daily
http://www.sciencedaily.com/releases/2010/03/100302171531.htm
Dysbiosis │ Wikipedia
http://en.wikipedia.org/wiki/Dysbiosis
Dysbacteriosis-Symptoms and Treatment │ Intestinal Dysbiosis
http://intestinaldysbiosis.com/dysbiosis/dysbacteriosis-symptoms-and-treatment
Gut flora │ Wikipedia
http://en.wikipedia.org/wiki/Gut_flora
WHFoods: vitamin K
http://www.whfoods.com/genpage.php?tname=nutrient&dbid=112
Coagulation │ Wikipedia
http://en.wikipedia.org/wiki/Coagulation
Cut Down on Sugar and Carbohydrates to Improve Health │ Natural News
http://www.naturalnews.com/023343_sugar_food_carbohydrates.html
Do Carbohydrates Turn To Sugar In Your Body? │ LIVESTRONG.COM
http://www.livestrong.com/article/505191-do-carbohydrates-turn-to-sugar-in-your-body/
Dietary Fiber │ Wikipedia
http://en.wikipedia.org/wiki/Dietary_fiber
Cruciferous vegetables │ Wikipedia
http://en.wikipedia.org/wiki/Cruciferous_vegetables

The Natural Path to Hormonal Wellness, Part 1 by Katarina Nolte
Pages: 201 (23,609 words); Copyright © 2014 by Katarina Nolte.
All rights reserved. http://katarinanolte.com/ July 2014

What are nightshades and in which foods are they found? | WHFoods

http://www.whfoods.com/genpage.php?tname=george&dbid=62

Insoluble fiber produces hard-to-pass stools that can distend and damage the intestinal lining, form blockages of compacted food, and create anal fissures. Excess soluble fiber creates massive fermentation and prodigious amounts of gases, acids, and alcohol, killing off the flora that normally hydrate stools and prevent constipation.

Negative Implications: Rethink the Role of Dietary Fiber | Natural News

http://www.naturalnews.com/029927_dietary_fiber_health.html

Flames

Fiber doesn't keep [the] "colon clean" by speeding elimination, according to the highly respected and authoritative Rome II: The Functional Gastrointestinal Disorders textbook: "There is little or no relationship between dietary fiber and whole gut transit time." In fact, fiber delays transit time more than does any other food ingredient, and is the primary cause of chronic constipation, hemorrhoids, diverticulosis, ulcerative colitis, and Crohn's disease.

Fiber Menace: The Truth About the Leading Role of Fiber in Diet Failure, Constipation, Hemorrhoids, Irritable Bowel Syndrome, Ulcerative Colitis, Crohn's Disease, and Colon Cancer

http://www.amazon.com/Fiber-Menace-Constipation-Hemorrhoids-Ulcerative/dp/0970679645/

When gastrointestinal health is compromised, the rest of the body doesn't work as it should.
Insoluble (indigestible) fiber ferments, forming gases, bloating, acidic wastes and intestinal inflammation, all of which disturb normal healing and regenerative processes.
If inflammation persists, becoming chronic, other imbalances occur, most frequently relating to blood sugar and insulin. Chronic inflammation leads to insulin resistance, which in turn causes diabetes, an exploding problem worldwide.
Chronic intestinal inflammation can cause belly fat accumulation (also related to blood sugar, insulin, diabetes, and cardiovascular problems) and depression, with researchers being unsure which

one comes first. What seems to be clear is that it all begins with chronic inflammation, which nowadays most commonly develops in the digestive tract. Further, excess weight compromises immunity, thereby prolonging inflammation. The primary cause of a chronically inflamed digestive system is stress in the form of mental and emotional stresses, and food, water, and air compromised by industry.

Type 2 Diabetes: Inflammation, Not Obesity, Cause of Insulin Resistance | Science Daily
http://www.sciencedaily.com/releases/2007/11/0711 06133106.htm
Human gastrointestinal tract | Wikipedia
http://en.wikipedia.org/wiki/Human_gastrointestinal_t ract#Immune_function
Diabetes becoming alarmingly common worldwide | Washington Post
http://www.washingtonpost.com/national/health-science/diabetes-becoming-alarmingly-common-worldwide-new-study-finds/2011/06/24/AGMkaFlH_story.html
Is Chronic Inflammation a Possible Cause of Obesity-Related Depression? | Hindawi
http://www.hindawi.com/journals/mi/2009/439107/
Inflammation | Wikipedia
http://en.wikipedia.org/wiki/Inflammation#Systemic_i nflammation_and_obesity
Gastrointestinal Diseases - Digestive System | Diet and Health
http://www.diet-and-health.net/Diseases/gastrointestinal.html

The Natural Path to Hormonal Wellness, Part 1 by Katarina Nolte
Pages: 201 (23,609 words); Copyright © 2014 by Katarina Nolte.
All rights reserved. http://katarinanolte.com/ July 2014

Uncomfortable digestive symptoms like bloating, gas, and bubbling in the gut arise because an overgrowth of yeast leads to the fermentation of foods instead of the digestion of foods. Along with these unpleasant symptoms, yeasts ferment sugars into alcohol, which destabilizes blood sugar and leads to intense cravings for more sugar. I find it fascinating that these tiny organisms can get us to do exactly what they want us to do — eat more carbs and sugar!

Yeast sensitivity, sugar cravings, and your digestion | Women to Women

http://www.womentowomen.com/digestionandgihealth/candida.aspx

Twist

Any health problems that compromise digestion and/or absorption of nutrients can contribute to deficiency of vitamin K. These problems include health conditions like inflammatory bowel disease, ulcerative colitis, celiac disease, short bowel syndrome, and digestive tract surgeries (like intestinal resection). Problems with pancreatic function, liver function, or gallbladder function can also increase our risk of vitamin K deficiency. Because our intestinal bacteria help supply us with vitamin K, any drugs that alter our normal intestinal bacteria can compromise our vitamin K status. At the top of this drug list would be antibiotics.
What factors might contribute to a deficiency of vitamin K? | WHFoods
http://www.whfoods.com/genpage.php?tname=nutrient&dbid=112

Disproportionate amounts of fiber jeopardize the digestion of vital proteins, fats, vitamins, minerals, and trace elements, with the effect being connective tissue weakness, musculoskeletal problems, neurological damage, etc.
Grains, high in fiber, gluten, lectins, and phytates, disturb the balance of both, the digestive and the hormonal system, resulting in food cravings, overeating, cellular damage, stomach lining damage, and the appearance of the by now well known digestive conditions like irritable bowel (IBS), inflammatory bowel (IBD), Celiac, Crohn's, Candidiasis, leaky gut (LGS), etc.

The Natural Path to Hormonal Wellness, Part 1 by Katarina Nolte
Pages: 201 (23,609 words); Copyright © 2014 by Katarina Nolte.
All rights reserved. http://katarinanolte.com/ July 2014

The main problem with high fiber foods is that they are not meant for human consumption because they are too difficult to impossible to digest and were therefore originally soaked, sprouted, fermented, and/or marinated, so as to be made somewhat edible in moderate amounts.
Unfortunately today, most people, regardless of where they live, use grains, corn, rice, and/or soy, as staple foods, thereby literally destroying their health and quality of life. To make matters worse, these and other foods are being increasingly genetically altered (GMOs) and exposed to poisonous substances originally invented to serve as weapons of war (pesticides, fungicides, herbicides, radiation, etc.).
As a result, children and adults suffer from the before mentioned digestive conditions along with, and related to malabsorption, malnutrition, autoimmune disease, and excess fat accumulations on and/or in the body (organ fat), with rotting, undigested food roaming freely and destroying vital organs and tissues.

The Lowdown On Lectins | Mark's Daily Apple
http://www.marksdailyapple.com/lectins/
Lectins | Wikipedia
http://en.wikipedia.org/wiki/Lectin
Essential Sugars and Plant Lectins | Failsafe Diet
http://failsafediet.wordpress.com/about-food-chemical-intolerance/the-natural-toxins-in-food/essential-sugars-and-plant-lectins/
Why No Grains and Legumes? Part 1: Lectins | Paleo Plan
http://www.paleoplan.com/2011/03-30/why-no-grains-and-legumes/

The Natural Path to Hormonal Wellness, Part 1 by Katarina Nolte
Pages: 201 (23,609 words); Copyright © 2014 by Katarina Nolte.
All rights reserved. http://katarinanolte.com/ July 2014

What are nightshades and in which foods are they found? │ WHFoods
http://www.whfoods.com/genpage.php?tname=george&dbid=62
FiberMenace: About the book │ Gut Sense
http://www.gutsense.org/fibermenace/about_fm.html
Cadaverine │ Wikipedia
http://en.wikipedia.org/wiki/Cadaverine
Diverticulosis and diverticulitis │ Gut Sense
http://www.gutsense.org/gutsense/diverticular.html
Why Grains Are Unhealthy │ Mark's Daily Apple
http://www.marksdailyapple.com/why-grains-are-unhealthy/#axzz1qa16Yvcq
Definitive Guide: The Primal Blueprint │ Mark's Daily Apple
http://www.marksdailyapple.com/definitive-guide-primal-blueprint/#axzz1qa16Yvcq

MAY I offer you some warm, bacteria-ridden dough topped with rotten milk and discs of rotten meat? No? That is a pepperoni pizza. If that sounds too unappetizing, substitute "bacteria-ridden" with "risen" (pizza crust, like bread, relies on the work of a unicellular fungus known as Saccharomyces cerevisiae—or, more commonly, yeast), and "rotten" with "fermented". The cheese and meat are both the delicious product of bacteria.
Fish sauce: The thin line between fermentation and rot │ Economist
http://www.economist.com/blogs/prospero/2011/05/fish_sauce

Flurry

Prior to fermented products such as soy sauce, tempeh, natto, and miso, soy was considered sacred for its use in crop rotation as a method of fixing nitrogen. The plants would be plowed under to clear the field for food crops.
Soybean History | Wikipedia
http://en.wikipedia.org/wiki/Soybean#History

Putrefaction (rotting) is done by microorganisms which impede digestion, nutrient absorption, and the elimination of wastes. Fermentation is done by microorganisms which support digestion, nutrient absorption, and the elimination of wastes.
Intentional fermentation has been practiced at least since the introduction of plant and animal domestication, and in particular since humans begun consuming grains, corn, rice, beans, soybean, lentils, and peas.
Fermentation extends the shelf life of food, intensifies the taste and aroma of food, and makes food easier to digest by increasing the amount of healthy gut bacteria (in the food itself and in the gut post consumption).
Examples of fermented foods are: raw fermented dairy products (yogurt, kefir, sour cream; fresh and aged cheeses), raw fermented vegetables (sauerkraut, pickles); raw fermented eggs, meat, fish or seafood (liver-, fish-, or shrimp pâté; fish-, or oyster sauce; mayonnaise); raw fermented nuts and seeds (raw vegan "cheeses", pâtés, and sauces), fermented grains (soured porridge, kashk, trahanas, dhokla, naturally fermented breads and

pastas), and fermented legumes (soy sauce, bean pâté, lactose-fermented lentils).

Constipation, as well as irritable bowel (IBS), inflammatory bowel disease (IBD), Crohn's, Candida, Celiac, leaky gut, etc., are all associated with insufficient amounts of friendly gut bacteria necessary for proper digestion. Therefore, naturally fermented foods may help some individuals replenish their flora.

Ideally, fermentation should be done at home, and one should stick with raw fermented foods, while avoiding grain-, soy-, and rice-based fermented foods and beverages.

Raw fermented foods offer a variety of flavors, are rich in enzymes, beneficial microorganisms, and vitamins, while cooking/pasteurization destroys them. Destruction of these vital substances, in turn, incapacitates the gut, exhausts the system, and leads to overall degeneration, including premature aging (example: adult diseases in children).

Fermented fruit is a high fiber, high sugar alcoholic product, be it edible or drinkable. It should not be consumed by people who are constipated, or those who suffer from digestive conditions like irritable bowel (IBS), inflammatory bowel disease (IBD), Crohn's, Candida, Celiac, leaky gut, etc.

Probiotics are helpful digestive probiotic bacteria for Crohns | Crohn's
http://www.crohns.net/Miva/education/whatprobiotics.shtml

181

More Evidence Links Gut Bacteria to Celiac Disease | Celiac
http://www.celiac.com/articles/21685/1/More-Evidence-Links-Gut-Bacteria-to-Celiac-Disease/Page1.html

Drunk Animals | Meta Cafe
http://www.metacafe.com/watch/90957/drunk_animals/

Poaceae | Wikipedia
http://en.wikipedia.org/wiki/Poaceae#Taxonomy

Cereal | Wikipedia
http://en.wikipedia.org/wiki/Cereal

Legume | Wikipedia
http://en.wikipedia.org/wiki/Legume

Difference Between Fermenting and Rotting | Super Foods for Super Health
http://www.superfoods-for-superhealth.com/Superfood_Evolution-fermented-food.html

Reflections on Rotten Food | Chow Hound
http://chowhound.chow.com/topics/286173

8 Reasons to Eat Fermented Foods | Cheese Slave
http://www.cheeseslave.com/got-bacteria-10-reasons-to-eat-fermented-foods/

Raw Ferments - The Missing Link - The Forgotten Superfood | Hidden Pond LLC
http://hiddenpondllc.com/content/4886

Injera | Wiki Books
http://en.wikibooks.org/wiki/Cookbook:Injera

Kashk | Wikipedia
http://en.wikipedia.org/wiki/Kashk

Tarhana | Wikipedia
http://en.wikipedia.org/wiki/Tarhana

Why We Love Lactofermentation | Cedar Circle Farm
http://cedarcirclefarm.org/tips/view/why-we-love-lactofermentation/

Would you eat fermented meat? | Paleo Hacks
http://paleohacks.com/questions/11937/would-you-eat-fermented-meat#axzz1sAVhZjOg
High vs. Fermented Meat | Raw Paleo Diet Forum
http://www.rawpaleodietforum.com/general-discussion/high-vs-fermented-meat/
Fermented Foods | Akea Life
http://www.akealife.com/blueprint-for-life/nutrition/fermented-foods/
Fermented Eggplant Recipe | Whole Traditions
https://www.wholetraditions.com/recipes/124-fermented-eggplant
Carciofi Sott'Olio: Marinated Artichokes Recipe | Food Network
http://www.foodnetwork.com/recipes/mario-batali/carciofi-sottolio-marinated-artichokes-recipe/index.html

Evidence has suggested that Dysbiosis plays a part in many conditions such as: Irritable Bowel Syndrome, Anklyosing Spondylitus, Rheumatoid Arthritis, Inflammatory Bowel Disease, Multiple Sclerosis, Chronic Fatigue, Eczema, food allergies. Many people are unaware that they are even suffering from Dysbiosis.
Dysbiosis and Leaky Gut Syndrome | Leaky Gut
http://www.leakygut.co.uk/Dysbiosis.htm

Fire

It is erroneous to assume that any evidence of fire from millennia ago, must be of human origin, and then further jump to conclude that humans have been cooking for millions of years.
Advent of Cooking | Raw Paleo Diet
http://www.rawpaleodiet.com/articles/dangers-of-cooked-foods-an-extensive-collection-of-on-and-offsite-articles/advent-of-cooking-article/

While natural fires in the form of volcanoes, lightning, and wildfires have been occurring over the past several hundred million years, research findings vary on the subject of when fire was first used by humans, and whether and when it has been used for the specific purpose of heating food. A similar disagreement exists on the question of when and how often humans created intentional fires, rather than taking advantage of accidental or natural fires on rare occasions.

It is, of course, also not known to what extent foods were cooked, whether they were lightly steamed, smoked, or seared, etc., or whether the food was boiled or roasted for extended periods of time. The importance of these details lies in the fact that most people today experience digestive problems with regular consumption of overcooked and/or over processed foods. If our ancestors would have been consuming overwhelmingly cooked foods, our digestive systems would have an easy time processing such foods.

On the other hand, humans are the only animals who heat their food, so perhaps an adaptation is

184

The Natural Path to Hormonal Wellness, Part 1 by Katarina Nolte
Pages: 201 (23,609 words); Copyright © 2014 by Katarina Nolte.
All rights reserved. http://katarinanolte.com/ July 2014

impossible. Pets which are fed mostly or exclusively processed foods (including foods cooked at home), tend to suffer from the same diseases as humans, when compared to pets whose diets consist of raw whole food (incl. bone, cartridge, internals, and outdoor plants, insects, etc.). The modern pet also tends to live half as long, on average.

Advent of Cooking | Raw Paleo Diet

http://www.rawpaleodiet.com/articles/dangers-of-cooked-foods-an-extensive-collection-of-on-and-offsite-articles/advent-of-cooking-article/

Socializing around a campfire might actually be an essential aspect of what makes us human.
Humans Used Fire 1 Million Years Ago | News | Discovery

http://news.discovery.com/human/human-ancestor-fire-120402.html

The Natural Path to Hormonal Wellness, Part 1 by Katarina Nolte
Pages: 201 (23,609 words); Copyright © 2014 by Katarina Nolte.
All rights reserved. http://katarinanolte.com/ July 2014

Jaws

*Our teeth are brachydont, and aren't intended for
chewing fiber, otherwise, after a decade or so, you
simply wouldn't have any teeth left to argue this
point with clarity. That's why the fiber for human
consumption is crushed, milled, or ground first, and
requires little or no chewing. But even after
processing, it affects the oral cavity with a menacing
vengeance.*

Fiber Menace: Excerpts from the book
http://fibermenace.com/fibermenace/fm_chapter1.htm
l

Parallel to the digestive tract being unable to
handle processed foods, human jaws and teeth
demonstrate the negative consequences of
processed food consumption. The human jaw first
shrunk when our archaic ancestors begun
processing food by hand, and then once again
since cooking was introduced, and again since the
introduction of grains into the diet. Some believe
that the shrinking of the human jaw, as well as the
teeth, is ongoing because of the industrial
revolution, the related spread of factory food
products, and the ever increasing availability of
portable, bite size food stuffs.
This means that over the past couple of million
years, humans reduced the frequency of biting into
food (fruit, bugs, meat, roots, whole animals),
followed by less chewing of raw foods (enzymes,
friendly bacteria, and other undenatured
nutrients), and a gradual increase in the amount of
grinding crunchy, chewy, sticky grain-based
products and processed grain-fed animal products.

186

The Natural Path to Hormonal Wellness, Part 1 by Katarina Nolte
Pages: 201 (23,609 words); Copyright © 2014 by Katarina Nolte.
All rights reserved. http://katarinanolte.com/ July 2014

As a result and unlike (other) animals, humans have jaws that often cannot accommodate all 32 teeth, which then are misaligned, maloccluded, and rotting away (caries), while the jaw degenerates (gingivitis, periodontitis). Studies show that tribal children outside of civilization tend to develop perfectly matching sets of teeth as long as they don't consume factory foods. If they do, a mismatched development of jaw size and shape relative to teeth size and shape occurs and is followed by decay, gum disease and tooth loss later in life.

Human 'dental chaos' linked to evolution of cooking | New Scientist
http://www.newscientist.com/article/dn7035
Dangers of Cooked Foods | Raw Paleo Diet
http://www.rawpaleodiet.com/articles/dangers-of-cooked-foods-an-extensive-collection-of-on-and-offsite-articles/
Toxins created by cooking | Raw Food Life
http://www.rawfoodlife.com/Articles___Research/Toxins_Created_by_Cooking/toxins_created_by_cooking.html
Epigenetics, DNA: How You Can Change Your Genes, Destiny | TIME.com
http://www.time.com/time/magazine/article/0,9171,1952313,00.html

The only body parts requiring regular surgery are the teeth.
Human 'dental chaos' linked to evolution of cooking | New Scientist
http://www.newscientist.com/article/dn7035

Brainy

Dietary fat is the only substance that initiates the action that precedes bowel movements.
Frequently Asked Questions: Constipation | Gut Sense
http://www.gutsense.org/constipation/faq.html

Between 3 million years ago and up until about 10,000-20,000 years ago, the average human brain increased in size in proportion to the increase in animal protein consumption (eggs, meat, seafood, fish, sea animals, and poultry). Among countless nutrients, the named animal products provided humans with high levels of healthy fats essential for thriving brains.

Presently it is known that inadequate amounts of healthy fats in the diet lead to an array of degenerative diseases, including serious digestive-, neurological- cardiovascular-, and musculoskeletal issues.

Toward the end of the last ice age, hunters ran out of game and began eating what basically amounts to indigestible grass seeds (grains).

Mass hunting involved enclosure, also known as corralling, during which hunters would surround large numbers of animals, and slaughter them as they moved inward into the center of the herd until all animals were dead. Eventually, instead of killing all animals, humans begun collecting the young, taming them by providing nutrition and safety, and animal domestication was born.

The Natural Path to Hormonal Wellness, Part 1 by Katarina Nolte
Pages: 201 (23,609 words); Copyright © 2014 by Katarina Nolte.
All rights reserved. http://katarinanolte.com/ July 2014

What followed was the consumption of domesticated plants and animals, which are of inferior nutritional quality when compared to wild plants and animals. The agricultural lifestyle required a previously unheard of workforce, which in turn lead to more offspring being produced. The combination of chronic malnutrition, excessive reproduction, resource based war, and socioeconomic stratification over the past 10,000 years caused the human brain (skull) and body to weaken and shrink.

The more recent industrial revolution changed this somewhat for the better, but overall, our ancestors like the archaic Homo Sapiens and Homo Sapiens Neanderthalensis continue to represent the most robust humans with the largest skulls to date.

Quaternary extinction event | Wikipedia
http://en.wikipedia.org/wiki/Quaternary_extinction_event

Civilization | Wikipedia
http://en.wikipedia.org/wiki/Civilization

If Modern Humans Are So Smart, Why Are Our Brains Shrinking? | Discover Magazine
http://discovermagazine.com/2010/sep/25-modern-humans-smart-why-brain-shrinking

Big Brain: The Origins and Future of Human Intelligence | Amazon
http://www.amazon.com/Big-Brain-Origins-Future-Intelligence/dp/1403979782

Neanderthals More Intelligent Than Thought | News | Discovery
http://news.discovery.com/history/neanderthals-more-intelligent-than-thought.html

All Non-Africans Part Neanderthal, Genetics Confirm | News | Discovery

http://news.discovery.com/human/genetics-neanderthal-110718.html
Asian Neanderthals, Humans Mated | News | Discovery
http://news.discovery.com/history/neanderthal-human-mating.html
Sex with Neanderthals Made Us Stronger | News | Discovery
http://news.discovery.com/human/neanderthals-interbreeding-humans-110825.html
Neanderthal Children Were Large, Sturdy | News | Discovery
http://news.discovery.com/history/neanderthal-baby-teeth-family.html
Neanderthal Males Had Popeye-Like Arms | News | Discovery
http://news.discovery.com/history/neanderthal-hormones-strong-arms.html
Advent of Cooking | Raw Paleo Diet
http://www.rawpaleodiet.com/articles/dangers-of-cooked-foods-an-extensive-collection-of-on-and-offsite-articles/advent-of-cooking-article/

Brain-size has decreased by 8% since the advent of the Agricultural Revolution, which coincided with a massive increase in the consumption of cooked starchy foods... An increase in cooked starches, grains and the introduction of dairy to the human diet, coupled with a decrease in meat has caused great detriment to our species.
Advent of Cooking | Raw Paleo Diet
http://www.rawpaleodiet.com/articles/dangers-of-cooked-foods-an-extensive-collection-of-on-and-offsite-articles/advent-of-cooking-article/

The Natural Path to Hormonal Wellness, Part 1 by Katarina Nolte
Pages: 201 (23,609 words); Copyright © 2014 by Katarina Nolte.
All rights reserved. http://katarinanolte.com/ July 2014

Captivity

Over the past 20,000 years, the average volume of the human male brain has decreased from 1,500 cubic centimeters to 1,350 cc, losing a chunk the size of a tennis ball. The female brain has shrunk by about the same proportion. If our brain keeps dwindling at that rate over the next 20,000 years, it will start to approach the size of that found in Homo erectus, a relative that lived half a million years ago and had a brain volume of only 1,100 cc.

If Modern Humans Are So Smart, Why Are Our Brains Shrinking? | Discover Magazine

http://discovermagazine.com/2010/sep/25-modern-humans-smart-why-brain-shrinking

The domestication of farm animals has lead to the domestication of humans themselves. Just like cattle and sheep, humans adapted by passing on decision making to whoever had power over food and food choices, the plain order of civilization. Instead of living in tiny close knit groups with no manmade territorial limits, humans now inhabited limited spaces with comparatively extremely large numbers of strangers. As a result, the autonomous independence of individuals living in the wild was replaced by duteous dependence of individuals living in a controlled environment. The artsy-craftsy skillfulness of the hunter-gatherer, or more accurately scavenger-gatherer-hunter, was fading and so was the human intellect. Normally, brain and body develop and grow in proportion, but at the onset of agriculture, the skull no longer grew to full completion, something that has been observed in domesticated animals as well. These new juvenile-brained humans favored reproduction with less aggressive (physically and otherwise), more compliant mates. As a result, the average lifespan dropped from 35 (pre-agricultural Paleolithic Era) to 25 (agricultural Greco-Roman Era), conservatively.

Neurodegenerative disease related to our grain-based diet and unnatural lifestyle affects the digestive tract as much as it affects the function and longevity of our brains. The consequence of agricultural civilization was not only the shrinking of the brain over generations, but also the shrinking and overall deterioration of the brain over the course of a lifetime.

Age related brain shrinkage begins around age 25 and is unique to the human species. Other animals (inc. primates) do not show such a decline, and it can therefore be concluded that the difference between us and other animals is the fact that we consume a diet to which we thus far have been unable to adapt to, and that as a consequence, we evolve, develop, and age in an inferior mode.

The Incredible Shrinking Human Brain | News | Science Mag
http://news.sciencemag.org/sciencenow/2011/07/the-incredible-shrinking-human-b.html
Our Brains Are Shrinking. Are We Getting Dumber? | NPR
http://www.npr.org/2011/01/02/132591244/our-brains-are-shrinking-are-we-getting-dumber
Nutrition for intellect | Daily Motion
http://www.dailymotion.com/video/xfqq52_nutrition-for-intellect_lifestyle

The Natural Path to Hormonal Wellness, Part 1 by Katarina Nolte
Pages: 201 (23,609 words); Copyright © 2014 by Katarina Nolte.
All rights reserved. http://katarinanolte.com/ July 2014

If Modern Humans Are So Smart, Why Are Our Brains Shrinking? | Discover Magazine
http://discovermagazine.com/2010/sep/25-modern-humans-smart-why-brain-shrinking
Rapid Uplift: Ancient People Were Smarter Than Us | Suvratk
http://suvratk.blogspot.com/2008/04/ancient-people-were-smarter-than-us.html
Big Brain: The Origins and Future of Human Intelligence | Amazon
http://www.amazon.com/Big-Brain-Origins-Future-Intelligence/dp/1403979782

In class today we examined the development of agriculture and compared hunter-gatherers to early Neolithic farmers. As humans domesticated plants and animals, the plants and animals themselves change over time. Wild sheep and mountain goats get fatter, slower, dumber, and lose their balance.
Learning to Farm | Mr Guerriero
http://mrguerriero.blogspot.com/2011/11/learning-to-farm.html

Denatured

I adhere to the philosophy that both the living organism and its enzymes are inhabited by a vital principle or life energy which is separate and distinct from caloric energy. The enzyme complex harbors a protein carrier inhabited by a vital energy factor.
Enzyme Nutrition by Dr. Edward Howell | Amazon
http://www.amazon.com/Enzyme-Nutrition-Dr-Edward-Howell/dp/0895292211/

When it comes to the gut, the brain, and other vitals, ORAC (Oxygen Radical Absorbance Capacity) levels in foods play a notable role. Some of the highest ORAC foods are berries, cacao, cloves, cinnamon, curry/turmeric, cumin, mustard, flax, chia, ginger, and culinary herbs. Industrially processed, cooked foods lack vital nutrients, and are more or less packed with artificial substances which the body has no use for, and which it is often unable to eliminate. Heating food over the maximum heating capacity of topsoil (115 °F/46°C) by the sun destroys enzymes, friendly bacteria (which causes mold to flourish), many vitamins, minerals, and trace elements. For this reason, industrially processed and/or overheated food has been given the term 'denatured' by people who consume foods with a focus on nutritional value, and enzyme activity in particular (raw-, paleo-, instinctive-, and local foodists, vegans, and vegetarians).
Denatured or 'dead' food tends to do the opposite of what food is supposed to do but can't without

the named nutrients. That is to nourish and cleanse the body. The repercussions of long term consumption of such foods are constipation and an accumulation of toxins for which the body builds up fat or tumors as storage spaces, as well as chronic diseases of the digestive tract and related organs, allergies, musculoskeletal- and cardiovascular problems, and autoimmune diseases (incl. AIDS).

Nutrition and Brain Function | Agricultural Research Service | USDA
http://www.ars.usda.gov/is/AR/archive/aug07/aging0807.htm
Top 100 High ORAC Value Antioxidant Foods | Modern Survival Blog
http://modernsurvivalblog.com/health/high-orac-value-antioxidant-foods-top-100/
Early dementia often caused by autoimmune disorders | Reuters
http://www.reuters.com/article/2008/04/15/us-early-dementia-often-caused-autoimmun-idUSPAT57989320080415
Autoimmune Causes of Dementia | Elaine Moore
http://elaine-moore.suite101.com/autoimmune-causes-of-dementia-a293654
Causes Of Early Onset Dementia | LIVESTRONG.COM
http://www.livestrong.com/article/118117-causes-early-onset-dementia/
How To Eat To Lose Weight | Heaven Ministries
http://www.heavenministries.com/health/how_to_eat_to_lose_weight_copyri.htm
Soil Temperature | Essortment
http://www.essortment.com/soil-temperature-54558.html
Review: Maximize Immunity (Comby) | Beyond Veg

The Natural Path to Hormonal Wellness, Part 1 by Katarina Nolte
Pages: 201 (23,609 words); Copyright © 2014 by Katarina Nolte.
All rights reserved. http://katarinanolte.com/ July 2014

http://www.beyondveg.com/nieft-k/rvw/rvw-maximize-immunity.shtml
Denaturation Protein | Elmhurst
http://www.elmhurst.edu/~chm/vchembook/568denaturation.html
How Can Constipation Function as a Root Cause of All Disease and Illness? | Health Begins in the Colon
http://www.healthbeginsinthecolon.com/chapter-summaries.html

"Sometimes I think my head is so big because it is so full of dreams," He might have been speaking for the Boskops, an almost forgotten group of early humans who lived in southern Africa between 30,000-10,000 years ago. The Boskops were similar to modern humans but had small, childlike faces and huge melon heads that held brains about 30% larger than our own.
The Extinct Human Species That Was Smarter Than Us | Discover Magazine
http://discovermagazine.com/2008/mar/21-the-extinct-human-species-that-was-smarter-than-us

The Natural Path to Hormonal Wellness, Part 1 by Katarina Nolte
Pages: 201 (23,609 words); Copyright © 2014 by Katarina Nolte.
All rights reserved. http://katarinanolte.com/ July 2014

Factory

Industrial agriculture also creates hunger and malnutrition at another level – by robbing crops of nutrients. Industrially produced food is a nutritionally 'empty mass', loaded with chemicals and toxins. Nutrition in food comes from the nutrients in the soil. Industrial agriculture, based on synthetic nitrogen –, phosphorus –, and potassium – based fertilisers, leads to the depletion of vital micronutrients and trace elements such as magnesium, zinc, calcium and iron.
Swaraj: A Deeper Freedom | Vandana Shiva
http://www.vandanashiva.org/?p=611

Modern industrial agriculture is operated by a small number of corporations and consists of Concentrated (or Confined) Animal Feeding Operations (CAFOs) and monocultural crop fields, biotech laboratories, agrochemical- and food factories; local-, state-, and international trade, and public relations, advertising, wholesale, and retail.

Agribusiness animals exist in conditions that are unsanitary and further deteriorate the quality of the resulting food. They are fed a mush consisting of genetically engineered grains, pharmaceuticals and other chemicals, plastic pellets (artificial roughage), rendered animal carcasses, manure/litter, blood, feathers, hairs and skins. Agribusiness plant foods are doused with pesticides, herbicides, fungicides, heavy metals, CAFO manure/litter, and artificial fertilizers.

Increasingly, fruits (incl. sugar cane), vegetables, fish, cattle, sheep, and goats are being genetically engineered and/or otherwise manipulated to reach specific criteria, most of which focus on short term profits rather than the quality of the product.
The quality of a food product is measured by its taste, aroma, and texture, all of which reflect its nutritional density. The nutritional density of a food product is dependent on the health of the soil, the water, the air, and the plant itself. In the case of animals, the nutritional quality of animal products depends on all of the above, as well as on the treatment of the animal by humans. To achieve superior food quality, farmers must be small scale, private, organic, and operating in ways that are as close to natural as possible, while accepting the fact that certain plants, animals, and sea creatures cannot be domesticated.
Ultimately, even if people lived in an environment that was completely free of industrial pollution, stress, and worry, industrial food alone would literally destroy their gastrointestinal function.

The Issues: Factory Farming | Sustainable Table
http://www.sustainabletable.org/issues/factoryfarming/
Factory Farms | Food and Water Watch
http://www.foodandwaterwatch.org/food/factoryfarms/
Living a Nightmare: Animal Factories in Michigan | Google Video
http://video.google.com/videoplay?docid=5163144866474931803
IS YOUR MEAT FIT TO EAT | Beyond Factory Farming
http://beyondfactoryfarming.org/files/BFF_Brochure07.pdf

How sustainable agriculture can address the environmental and human health harms of industrial agriculture | ncbi.nlm.nih.gov
http://www.ncbi.nlm.nih.gov/pmc/articles/PMC1240832/

The Meatrix
http://www.themeatrix.com/

Agrochemical | Wikipedia
http://en.wikipedia.org/wiki/Agrochemical

Agriculture | Wikipedia
http://en.wikipedia.org/wiki/Agriculture

Industrial agriculture (crops) | Wikipedia
http://en.wikipedia.org/wiki/Industrial_agriculture_(crops)

Monoculture | Wikipedia
http://en.wikipedia.org/wiki/Monoculture

They Eat What? The Reality of Feed at Animal Factories | Food & Agriculture | Union of Concerned Scientists
http://www.ucsusa.org/food_and_agriculture/science_and_impacts/impacts_industrial_agriculture/they-eat-what-the-reality-of.html

Genetically modified food | Wikipedia
http://en.wikipedia.org/wiki/Genetically_modified_food

GMO Fruit Facts | Youtube
http://www.youtube.com/watch?v=-qCS19sK6h0

Talking Fruit: How To Tell If Fruit Is Genetically Modified | Plantea
http://www.plantea.com/genetically-modified-foods.htm

Seven Deadly Myths of Industrial Agriculture | eHow
http://www.ehow.com/about_5195502_seven-deadly-myths-industrial-agriculture.html

Why Agriculture? | Nashville Urban Harvest
http://nashvilleurbanharvest.org/pages/why-get-involved-in-agriculture

The Natural Path to Hormonal Wellness, Part 1 by Katarina Nolte
Pages: 201 (23,609 words); Copyright © 2014 by Katarina Nolte.
All rights reserved. http://katarinanolte.com/ July 2014

Exploring the Link Between Animal Health and Food Safety | Food Safety News
http://www.foodsafetynews.com/2012/05/exploring-the-link-between-animal-health-and-food-safety/

Raj Patel Discusses Stuffed & Starved | Raj Patel
http://rajpatel.org/2009/11/11/raj-patel-discusses-stuffed-starved/

Genetic Chile | Vimeo
http://vimeo.com/11416802

How can you keep kosher when your rice pudding has human DNA in it? | OpEdNews.com
http://www.opednews.com/articles/GMOs-and-JEWS---Muslims-by-Linn-Cohen-Cole-090211-386.html

FRESH the movie
http://www.freshthemovie.com/

When we examine how our food is grown today, it becomes clear that most of the chemical tools taken for granted by modern agribusiness are products of warfare. Is this merely an indirect consequence of the tragic history of the 20th century, or does it suggest that the currently dismal state of our soils, fresh water supplies and rural economies is an outgrowth of agribusiness emergence from wartime in some important ways? Virtually all of the leading companies that brought us chemical fertilizers and pesticides made their greatest fortunes during wartime. How can this help us understand the ever-deteriorating quality of mass produced food?

Agribusiness, Biotechnology and War | Social Ecology
http://www.social-ecology.org/2002/09/agribusiness-biotechnology-and-war/

This was the first chapter from my book "So Long Constipation, Part 1". "So Long Constipation, Part 1" is available in paperback, ebook, and audiobook format everywhere where books are sold.